I0410440

There is **NO** HEALTH Pill!
Secrets to Getting Off or Avoiding
Prescription Drugs and Reclaiming True Health.

by

Scott duPont

Introduction by
Felicia Stoler, DCN, MS, RDN, FACSM, FAND
America's Health & Wellness Expert®

First Edition

This book is to be read by any person of any age and at any level of health or sickness with results of improved health, vitality, and increased energy. Just like life the more you put into it, the more you will get out of it. Hope you enjoy!

There is **NO** HEALTH Pill!
Secrets to Getting Off or Avoiding
Prescription Drugs and Reclaiming True Health.

Released and Published by:

Nemours Publishing
c/o Nemours Marketing, Inc.
7531 Azurebrook Court
Winter Park, FL 32792
Tel: (407) 738 - 1608

There is **NO** HEALTH Pill!
www.TheHealthPill.com
ISBN # 978-1540799654

U.S.	$16.99
Canada	$19.49

Other Health Books by Scott duPont

A Smoothie a Day Keeps the Doctor Away:
The Beginning
(Contributing Author)

Buttered Popcorn For Your Soul: Kernels of Inspiration,
Humor and Truth from Hollywood's Dreamers and Doers
(Contributing Author)

Do These Things or You Will Die
5 Secrets to a Long, Healthy, & Energetic Life!
(Author)

The Book of Inspiring & Thought Provoking
CANCER Quotes
(Author)

The Book of Inspiring & Thought Provoking
HEALTH Quotes
(Author)

Acknowledgements

Although this book took 2 years to finally put together, it was really a 10 + year journey in the making including my foray into the pharmaceutical world. First I'd like to thank Tracy Frenkel who cast me in my very first industrial video for Novartis and a few years later Julia Denton who introduced me to the Medco world. Thanks to Dr. Allan Konopacki for seeking me out on the floor of the American Academy of Family Physicians convention and it was an honor to work with you and Jonathan Jedd for several years. Of course a big thank you to Venetta Scott – my super agent who booked me on hundreds of health benefit fairs around the country for Express Scripts and who also managed to keep track of all the different cities, flights, hotels, etc. during many hectic open enrollment seasons.

To all the Human Resource people and the Health Care Benefits managers who allowed me to come into your world including Mark Tyndall. People like you really care about the health and well being of 'your people'. Not everyone sees all the time and effort you invest to deliver good health benefits despite the challenges of rapidly rising heathcare and drug costs every year.

Once again, a huge thank you to my friend Tony Robbins. Tony, through all of your detailed research and interviews with world-renowned doctors and experts of this subject, you really enlightened me on some profound tools to get healthier. You lit a fire in me to research the power of alkalinity even more and I've been sharing this info with as many people as possible. You are one of the most altruistic people I've ever met and I applaud all the lives you've touched and changed for the better including my own.

Thank you to the hundreds of people who trusted me to go through the 7-Day "Alkalize & Energize" cleanse program and give detailed feedback. I also appreciate all those folks willing to share your amazing results including: Bruce Ellington, Ronald Farnham, Andrew Reilly, Vanessa Esperanza, Desmond Bailey, Peter Allport, Andrew Diodati, Phil & Willie Jones and countless others

Thanks to Aleksandra Kyoseva for being the very first interview for the documentary film version of this book. I appreciate your candidness about your sickness created by your new American diet having moved here just a few years prior from Romania.

Thank you as well to my research team at Nemours Marketing, Inc. including Scott Townsend. Even your work part-time has been a huge help with this project.

To Josh Laronge, Once again I appreciate your creative genius with coming up with the cool Health Pill artwork design. Congratulations on your improved health and weight loss as well!

To the numerous Medco and Express customers over the last two decades who volunteered your incredible stories about how you (or your family members) got off of prescriptions, beat cancer or reclaimed your health. These inspirational stories clearly demonstrated to me that alternative, holistic therapies starting with excellent nutrition and daily exercise programs can work wonders!

To those Express Scripts customers not taking any daily prescriptions who I describe in this book as the *"Super Healthy 4%."* Your willingness to share so candidly your excellent daily habits and traits (which you all have in common) was so inspiring. I share your common daily habits at the end of the book, which I hope thousands of people will also embrace. You all are truly the 'poster children' for perfect health!

To my publicist Bill Hooey, Thanks in advance for helping spread the word about this book. Whether the message in this book helps hundreds, thousands or millions of people over time reclaim their excellent health, I know it can be done with your help in getting this important information out.

Thanks always to my trusted legal council Nicole Weaver. You are truly a 'Legal Eagle' with all the help and excellent advice you've provided over the years.

To Monroe Mann, Nicole Abisinio, and Marla Grosslight for giving me the time to do extended interviews which will give people a lot of insight on how to make their own worlds a little bit happier and healthier.

To Dr. Larry Oexner and Kim Oexner. Keep up all the great work you're doing at Urban Health and thanks for your help with some of the initial "Health Pill" live event tour stops we did in Florida. I hope we can do some more in the future. A big thanks also to Bruce Timmons for helping get the tour off the ground last year and all the other support staff who worked so hard.

A last minute thank you to Steve Harrison and Bradley Communications for your excellent advice over the years, including Martha Bullen for your great notes right before going to press!

Finally, I'd like to thank Nick Yaya for not only sharing your great story, but once again for your help going through the entire book to make my grammar and punctuation look a lot better. I look forward to really celebrating with you at the Academy Awards in a year or two.

Thank you all who are now reading this book!

Scott duPont

TABLE OF CONTENTS

Legal Disclaimer

There's NO guarantee the information in this book will improve your health and/or well being, but it is the author's belief that understanding (and most importantly) <u>applying</u> the numerous principles in the book "may help" you live a longer, healthier, and more energetic life.

This book is NOT intended to replace any medical advice or supersede your doctor's specific instructions, especially those individuals taking prescription drugs or under specific care of any medial professional(s). While there are references to several people I've worked with who are no longer taking prescription drugs or who have opted not to follow 'traditional' treatments or surgical options, I can't advise you to follow suit. The examples and specific people referenced in the book who have gotten off their prescriptions worked closely with their doctors to wean off their medications only after they started showing clear improvements to their health.

This book is NOT an expose about doctors, the medical field, or the pharmaceutical industry, as they all have their proper place. Rather this book will introduce many ideas based upon the long-standing doctrine *"Prevention is the Best Medicine"*. It is recommended that ANY alteration of your prescription drug regimen, or the implementation of any diet or exercise program be done with the consultation of a licensed medical, nutritional, or exercise professional.

If after reading this book you feel that the information that follows did NOT help you become healthier in any way, or you did not like the contents of this book, simply send back the book for a full refund under Nemours Marketing's 100% Total Satisfaction Guarantee as spelled out at the end of this book.

Foreword: There is NO Health Pill!

If we're HONEST with ourselves, we know that there is NO magic 'Health Pill' as much as we all want one for whatever health issues we may have. My name is Scott duPont and I'm not a doctor, I'm not a pharmacist and never went to medical school. Why in God's name would anyone read a health book about prescription drugs (or how to get off them specifically) from someone without the proper credentials? Before I answer that, I need to emphasize that I have the greatest respect for medical doctors and pharmacists who work in the most advanced heath care system in the world we have here in the U.S. I believe most doctors and pharmacists deeply care about their patients and do their best to serve them given the time and financial constraints within our flawed system.

So what is my background? I started out as pre-Medicine in college and although I did not pursue that field, I've always been fascinated with biology, anatomy, physiology and as long as I remember had an interest in health and fitness. Fast forward a few decades later, and I'm a working actor occasionally in scrubs on TV shows like "Gray's Anatomy" or "Code Black". However, I more often get hired by pharmaceutical companies to host corporate training videos and live events at medical conventions. Almost fifteen years ago, I got hired by Medco - a large pharmacy benefits manager (PBM) to give presentations and answer basic questions people have at health benefit fairs. (A side note: Medco is not a pharmaceutical company and does not manufacture or sell any drugs. As a PBM, Medco is the 'administrator' that allows consumers to get the prescriptions they need from the drug companies either at the retail pharmacy or through the mail). These health fairs take place during the 'open enrollment period' which for most corporations is October or November. I get hired to travel around the country and help a lot of confused people about how to save money on their prescriptions (through generics, mail order or alternative prescription drugs), answer questions, and as 'the front line messenger' listen to any concerns and help resolve them. When I first started working with Medco, my presentations were pretty simple and no longer than 5 minutes. It's steady work for an actor and I like the gigs and truly enjoy helping people. About 4 or 5 years ago, Medco merged with Express Scripts to become the largest PBM in the US. The merger of the two companies followed by an acquisition of Accredo (a large and well respected Specialty pharmacy) created incredible resources that better help the end customers get the proper prescriptions, save money, and help navigate the confusing maze of the highly complex drugs for advanced disease states including cancer. I was trained by Medco before I started my first gig and have done numerous training sessions and Teleconferences with Express Scripts over the years, and have learned so much by being at hundreds of these health fairs.

The genesis for this book was when I started to see some very disturbing trends (especially in the last few years). I started to see many more young people in their 20s and 30s taking multiple prescription drugs every day. I also began started encountering individuals at health fairs who were taking over 20 different prescriptions a day. Depending upon how many pills and how many doses prescribed, that can easily be 40 to 60 pills a day! The people I see at these health benefits fairs seem to be getting sicker. I've noticed more people taking blood pressure and cholesterol medications, but most alarming in the last 3 years, I've seen a huge increase in the number of people who are diabetic and/or have cancer. One indication of this disturbing trend was that my initial 5 minute presentation I gave a few years ago has now been expanded into a presentation that can run 30 minutes! I spend a lot more time addressing the mail-order program (since more people now are on 'daily' maintenance prescriptions), the myriad of specialty and cancer therapies, as well as the new mobile app, since managing prescription drugs has become a daily task for many people. The bright spot of every health fair is not only the people I'm able to help (which is nice), but the small group of people I encounter who seem to have absolutely perfect health. In the book, I call these people the "Super Healthy 4%" as approximately 4% of all the people I see on an average day are these vivacious, energetic people who often look 10 to 20 years younger than their actual age.

They take no prescriptions or over-the-counter drugs. I became obsessed with learning the secrets these people shared with me over the last 15 years. After listening to all these people and studying them, I found it interesting that they all shared almost identical daily habits, disclosed at the end of this book. I was in this strange world of witnessing people - sometimes the very same people year after year (as I have clients such as the State of New Mexico Retirees I've worked with the past three years getting older and sicker right before my eyes), yet at the same time I'd occasionally see a few of my "*Super Healthy 4%*" friends who seemed not to age a day. Then of course, there's all the public information about the sad state of our healthcare system. You don't have to work in this industry to realize that people in the U.S. are getting fatter, sicker, taking more prescriptions then ever, and more prone to diseases and cancer. It's impossible for anyone not to notice the skyrocketing healthcare costs including insurance co-pays and the rising cost of prescription drugs. I often get worried for my clients (both the employers and the employees) and how this expensive healthcare epidemic is going to end up. The Affordable Care Act promised to lower insurance premiums by $2,500 a year, offer more doctor choices, and allow access for everybody to quality healthcare and affordable prescription drugs. Things have not worked out as planned and I don't want to be overly pessimistic, but from what I see on the front lines (especially with so many more people addicted to expensive prescription drugs), it will take a miracle to fix our system. The whole medical system is broken and might soon be broke. I wrote my first health book over 5 years ago: Do These Things or You Will Die... 5 Secrets to a Long, Healthy, & Energetic Life! because I'd lost almost a dozen family members and close friends in a few short years to cancer and other lethal diseases. I felt compelled and inspired to write this new book, because even though I can't fix the system, I can offer YOU a potential solution for YOUR own health: a detailed plan with a plethora of information I've learned over the last 15 years on how to reclaim your health.

Getting back to the question of why listen to me vs. a medical doctor or pharmacist? The average doctor spends 8 to 9 years in school and many more years in residency before he or she can treat patients on their own. Almost all of their education is focused on traditional treatments including surgery and or prescription drug therapies. Most medical doctors spend less than two weeks studying nutrition and/or physical fitness and they are NEVER taught how to get people off prescriptions. Pharmacists can also spend 8 years in school and many spend decades later in pharmacies studying thousands of different prescription drugs as well as the hundreds of new drugs and all over-the-counter remedies. Most are incredibly knowledgeable about how all the drugs work and understanding the possible side effects and interactions. On the other hand, I've spent my whole life interested in physical fitness and nutrition and have read and studied hundreds of books on these subjects. Being around the pharmaceutical industry and interacting with thousands of people taking prescription drugs, I've noticed what is NOT working. If we measure success by how 'healthy' our population is in the U.S., the results are abysmal! This book is NOT an expose of big pharma or prescription drug pricing even though many people have a right to be upset about increasing drug prices. This book is about solutions and what YOU can do yourself to improve your health so you don't need to take as many (or hopefully any) daily prescriptions. Over the years, I obsessively asked questions like "How can I have more natural energy?", "How can I be even healthier?", "How can I avoid getting sick?". There's a lot more to my background I'll share in this book including many clients I've helped lose weight, reclaim their health, and in many cases gotten off all their prescription drugs. Not to brag, but at some of my "HEALTH Pill" live seminars and events, people often loiter around for an hour or so to chat and to thank me for unique information and health strategies they've never been exposed to before. While the typical pharmacist has been studying the myriad of new drugs coming to market and what diseases they can treat, I've been studying the healthiest, most energetic people in the world and learning what makes them stay fit and healthy. I'm always seeking the best and fastest ways to get other people healthier and most importantly, I look for long term, proven RESULTS.

Most of the information in this book might seem mundane, some you might have heard before, and frankly a few 'know it alls' might get bored with the book and want your money back. That's fine... turn to the last page of this book and you'll find instructions to get a complete refund. What I'm hoping for is that you will give me the benefit of the doubt to read the first few chapters and apply some of the information you've learned (or perhaps knew already, but weren't applying). I've specifically put together ACTION ITEMS at the end of every chapter. Often times we know what to do to improve our health, but until we understand the psychology behind *WHY* we're motivated to make some changes, and until we APPLY the information we learn, nothing changes. For the 39 different Action Items, you'll notice that they are very quick and easy to do. If you apply even just a few of the concepts and strategies in this book, I know in my heart you will reclaim your health. Everyone's health situation is different as some people might lose 20 pounds while others might lose 100. Some people might get off all of their prescription drugs while others might get off a few of their prescriptions and simply feel a lot better. Whatever your specific situation, I wish you all the best and if you end up having a health success story to share, please let me know. You have no idea what it means to me to me to hear the good news of someone reclaiming their health.

One final note, if you like the book and would like to see a copy donated to your child's school, your local library or your alma mater, please let me know. I'm donating hundreds of books to schools and libraries where they can make a difference for others. I'm also doing free live events around the country and if you'd like to attend, visit www.TheHealthPill.com for details. A final disclosure, at this point in time I have NO financial interests in any of the health or fitness products, tools, apps, nutritional supplements, etc. mentioned in this book. I only endorse quality products I believe can truly make a difference in your health. There are many people and companies selling expensive products and pricy supplements that in reality don't work very well or simply give you expensive urine. Many of the products, foods, supplements mentioned in the book you can get at your local store, grocery, or farmer's market.

Cheers to your perfect health!

Scott

PS - If you like the book or if it helped you in any way, please write a review on Amazon or where ever you purchased it. We don't have a large advertising budget and depend on 'word of mouth' for this book to get out and help as many people as possible. Thank you...

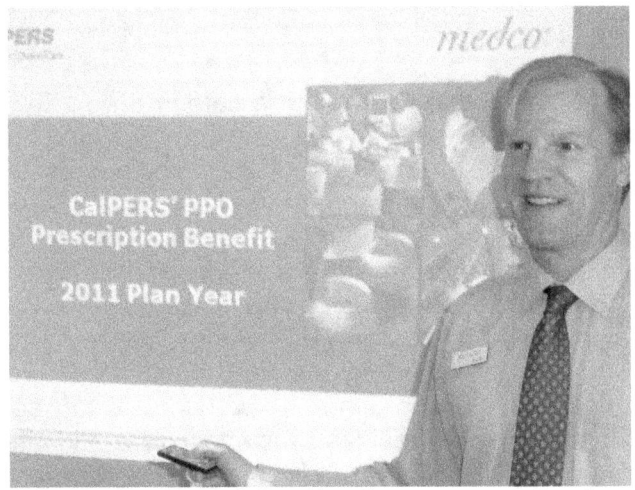

The author Scott duPont hosting a presentation for
Medco at a health benefits fair.

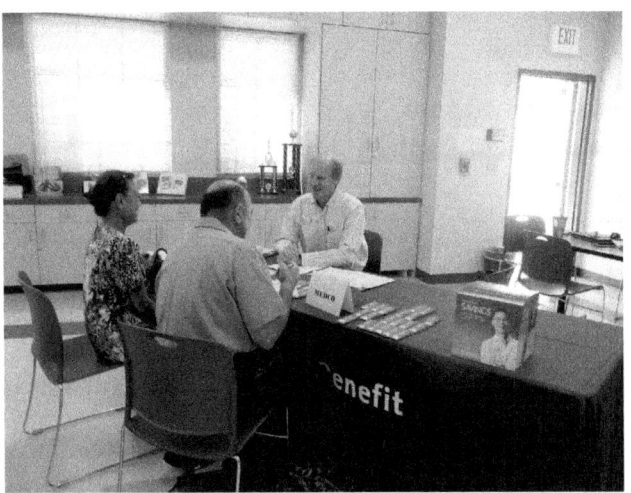

Educating a couple about their maintenance
prescriptions and mail order options.

Introduction

The first time I met Scott was at a café in Studio City, CA and we seemed to have quite a bit in common starting with being from the Garden State of New Jersey. Scott was very fit and exuded amazing energy, but more impressive was his passion for helping people regain optimum health. It's similar to the passion that I share all the time, from book, news interviews, speaking engagements to the television show I hosted on TLC: "Honey, We're Killing the Kids!" It was intriguing to me that Scott came from a pharmaceutical background - working with several prescription drug companies; and most recently with the two largest pharmacy benefit managers (Medco and Express Scripts). I agree 1000% with Scott's message that as a society, we often are too quick to blame our own health demise on our 'bad genes', and many prefer to reach for another 'pill' to fix our health problems.

Scott's 'big picture' message in his newest book is that we didn't just wake up one day 20 lbs. overweight, end up with Type 2 diabetes suddenly after a few bad meals, or abruptly lack energy after our 50th birthday. Most of us let our health slip due lifestyle choices: busy work schedules, not exercising properly while trying to keep up with our families and kids, while hoping to navigate the confusing food choices (many which are NOT healthy) in today's culture. I have to admit I was in your shoes about 20 years ago when I was working 50 to 70 hours per week at a large law firm in Manhattan. I let my drive for work, being "single in the city", and learning how to live on my own take precedent over my priority to maintain a healthy lifestyle. It took shopping for a bridesmaid dress for my younger sister's wedding to be my wake up call. My clothing size doubled as I was 20 lbs. overweight, I was mortified. I tried every diet in the magazines, got bad advice from the trainers at the gym and eventually ended up seeing a registered dietitian. She changed my life... so much so that I decided to change careers and become a registered dietitian nutritionist and exercise physiologist. I initially blamed my demise on my 'fat genes' until I began studying the science of nutrition, movement and human physiology.

Not only did I change my own life, but it became my life's mission to help and educate others. Scott's solution to all this madness is common sense:

1) Most of us are not getting our daily dose of fruits and veggies, and there is NO pill or potion or super food that can replace what we should be eating daily. Scott offers easy to follow tips to change your diet.

2) Many of us don't have extra time after work to drive to the gym and work out. You don't have to because this book lays out dozens of simple, easy-to-implement exercise strategies that anyone can squeeze into their busy lifestyle! Scott lays out a healthy, active *lifestyle* even the busiest executive or multi-tasking mom can embrace.

3) Scott explores the psychology of the people he observed as the "Super Healthy 4%". He takes you inside the minds of hundreds of healthy, happy people he encountered at health benefit fairs who exude a positive, optimistic outlook and clearly explains the mind-body connection.

In my first book: Living Skinny in Fat Genes®: The Healthy Way to Lose Weight and Feel Great, I shared many useful tips, ideas and healthy recipes so that readers could take action. Similarly, after each chapter in this book, Scott offers simple, easy to implement 'Action Items' that will serve as stepping stones towards reclaiming the excellent health you deserve.

I'm living proof that you can live skinny (and healthy) with whatever genes you inherited from your family. If you embrace the principles Scott lays out in this book, you too can lose unwanted weight, get off some of your prescription drugs, and reclaim the energy you had many years ago. This is not a 'get healthy quick' scheme, but a common sense approach that has worked for Scott and hundreds of others (many of their incredible stories are revealed in this book). If you embrace Scott's simple, realistic, and attainable changes in your daily habits, over time you will see impressive results. My very best wishes for a healthier and happier life!

Felicia Stoler, DCN, MS, RDN, FACSM, FAND
America's Health & Wellness Expert®

SECTION I:
The Fuel (Food) You Put in Your Tank

"The food you eat can be either the
safest and most powerful form of
medicine or the slowest form of poison."
- Ann Wigmore

Chapter 1.
The Bureau of Alcohol, Tobacco, Firearms and Explosives

The first time I heard 'The Bureau of Alcohol, Tobacco, and Firearms' (the bureau now includes explosives), was the opening monologue by a Las Vegas comedian. The comedian rambled on for several minutes about the absurdity of "someone getting really drunk, lighting up a cigarette and then picking up a gun... what a great combination!". He went on about the bureaucracy of different government agencies that have been grouped together for no logical reason. By the end of his ATF skit, I was laughing so hard he had me in tears. Even though it's humorous how the U.S. government operates sometimes, honestly these items: alcohol, tobacco and firearms do not belong together at all! Perhaps alcohol and tobacco together is logical, and a government agency grouping firearms and explosives makes sense, but the way the bureau groups all these items together today makes no sense. So, what does The Bureau of Alcohol, Tobacco, Firearms and Explosives have to do with health? It is purely a metaphor of government agencies and bureaucracy that were probably created with the best of intentions many decades ago, but make no sense today. So here's the huge problem our government has created that doesn't work today as the famous health expert and author Michael Pollan described on a recent Teleseminar: "We have no national 'Food' Policy', but rather an 'Agricultural' Policy". The Food and Drug Administration (FDA) policy set in place decades ago gives massive subsidies to corn and soybean growers with a large portion of these crops being GMO or genetically modified organisms. Much of the corn goes towards artificial sweeteners and fillers while a large portion of the soy goes into soy oil (an inexpensive oil used in a lot of processed and fast foods). However, 60% of the corn and 47% of the soy produced in the US is not being consumed by people, but by livestock! [1-1] These subsidized, super-cheap crops are supplemented by massive amounts of antibiotics to grow the chickens, hogs, cattle and other animals in factory farms at unprecedented rates. In fact, 80% of the antibiotics sold in the U.S. are used on mostly healthy animals on factory farms.[1-2] My hat's off to the government policy makers, farmers, scientists, chemists, and pharmaceutical companies as they have achieved and/or surpassed their goal to make super-cheap, well-preserved corn and soy based food that can be delivered to the masses. The US also has the most efficient, high volume and low priced meat and dairy products in the world that feed our population more meat and dairy per capita than any other nation on the planet. Now I'm not denouncing fast food on occasion, but there are many problems with consuming the amount of these processed corn and soy products as well as the abundance of meat Americans carve up every day. Even if you ignore the animal cruelty in many of these factory farms (increasingly caught on video), the massive environmental damages created, and the poor use of valuable resources (such as water) to grow many of these crops and livestock, the real problem in relation to this health book is that the government (via the FDA) is essentially subsidizing (or involuntarily promoting) millions of cases of Type II diabetes, heart disease, and cancer every year! In some of the other chapters ahead, I'll reference beyond any shadow of a doubt how these low cost processed foods, meats and dairy products are creating more and more health problems, which keep pushing the envelope of our trillion dollar healthcare industry! Americans spend hundreds of billions of dollars on doctor visits and surgeries each year, but the scary cost is that the U.S. spent almost $374 billion on prescription drugs alone in 2014, a 13% increase from the year before.[1-3] Being on the front lines every year at the Express Scripts table, I'm seeing a significant increase in younger people (in their 20's and 30's) taking daily 'maintenance' prescriptions or injecting insulin for their newly acquired diabetes. More medical professionals are now admitting that Type II diabetes, obesity, heart disease, and many cases of cancer could be reversed or minimized by getting the majority of our population off this cheap, non-healthy food diet. Here's a real world example of the Government (bureaucratic) problem I see at the grocery store every single day. Last night I was in a long line at my local Jons Grocery store getting ready to pay for my basket of fresh vegetables and fruits while the person in front of me pulled out their food stamp card (a fancy looking EBT debit card) paid for courtesy of the taxpayers. The morbidly obese lady in front of me (she probably weighed 300 lbs.) flanked by her two kids (both of them were at least 10 to 20 lbs. overweight) started unloading her bounty onto the conveyer belt which included two boxes of sugar-ladened cereal, Pop Tarts, Eggo frozen waffles, a 12-pack of Diet Coke, several 2-liter bottles of Pepsi, frozen Tater Tots, six frozen dinners, a large package of frozen hamburgers, a small package of hot dogs, etc. (I think you get the point). Now I'm not here to judge anyone, as it can be a challenge to feed a family on a limited budget even with $400.00 in monthly food stamps. However, ALL of these processed, sugary foods along with cheap meat and dairy products are creating health problems that our government subsidized health care later will be paying for the rest of their lives! The cost for heart disease, including surgery, can easily run over $100,000.00. But let's take a closer look at one of this lady's children in front of me in the grocery line. This young boy (who was chomping down on a Milky Way candy bar) I estimated to be ten years old and looked to be at least 20 lbs. overweight. God forbid this poor child gets Type II diabetes...according to the American Diabetes Association (ADA) website, the high cost of treatment are from expenditures including: hospital inpatient care (43% of the total medical cost), prescription medications to treat complications of diabetes (18%), anti-diabetic agents and diabetes supplies (12%), physician office visits (9%), and nursing/residential facility stays (8%). The average cost of medical expenditures for people with diabetes according to the ADA is $13,700.00 per year.[1-4] If this ten year old is lucky and lives to be 65, that's 55 years of treatment which would equal $753,500.00! And that's not adjusting for inflation or taking into account the exponential rising costs of medical treatment every year (the ADA saw a 41% increase over a five year period ending in 2012)! Now if this child doesn't climb above the median income level, he could either get all or part of his future medical expenses once again subsidized by the taxpayers! These insane, massive government subsidies for processed foods (especially corn and corn based sweeteners) are making millions of people sick and diseased every year and then ultimately leading to millions of people who then receive government subsidies or free healthcare treatment and prescription drugs! I'm not sure that the Bureau of Alcohol, Tobacco, Firearms and Explosives makes sense, but I know that this is an outdated FDA Policy that is adding to our current and future Health Care Crisis. These are staggering costs that individuals, corporations, and our government will not be able to pay in the coming years, especially if medical costs keep rising much faster than the adjusted inflation rate. It should be common sense that sooner or later the bank to pay for all of these sick people will run out of funds. It's time to come up with a sensible National Food Policy. When I speak at health seminars, often someone in the audience will ask: "So Scott, if you were in charge of the Government's Health Policy, what would you do? Do you have a solution?". I'm glad when that question gets asked because I have an answer. Over time (perhaps over 5 to 10 years) I'd begin phasing out these massive subsidies contributing to unhealthy, processed foods. I would immediately place a small sugar or 'junk food' tax on these unhealthy foods. Especially sodas and candy in the case where a single soda bottle or one candy bar exceeds the recommended daily allowance for sugar intake! Perhaps a 1 to 2-cent tax the first year, a 3-cent tax the second year, and then slowly keep raising this cost over time, which would eventually change consumer behavior. One of the things that worked successfully to lower tobacco use (which we also know causes cancer and lung disease, etc.) is that along with better warning labels and advertisements over the years, was the large tax placed on cigarettes. The increased taxes over time significantly reduced demand for cigarettes especially among teenagers and young adults. My proposed junk food tax would work the same way. Another thing I'd do is not necessarily cut food stamp benefits - as tens of millions of people, including many working full-time at minimum wage jobs truly need these benefits to feed themselves and their families, but I'd put some restrictions on these junk food products. Since America is a free country, I'd never tell people what food they can or cannot buy. If people want to buy cigarettes, liquor, or junk food with their own money, that's their personal right; but the taxpayers (you, me, and everyone else paying taxes) should NOT be subsidizing these sugar-laden junk foods that make people sick! There could be another easy fix with all the food stamp cards I often see being used at my local grocery store. My other idea would be to create a UPC code that denies payment for certain unhealthy items like sodas or candy. I saw a great example of how these codes work the other day - a gentleman at the same Jons Grocery store tried to sneak a $6.00 bottle of wine in along with all his other groceries. The register scanner beeped and read 'ineligible', so this man had $30.79 of his other groceries paid for by his EBT card, but he then had to cough up $6.00 of his own money for his bottle of wine. If we set up codes for certain high risk junk foods (like sodas, candy, etc), that would be a great incentive not to eat as much junk food. I'm not saying that people can't keep drinking soda or eating their favorite candies, but under my program the most extremely high health-risk foods like certain sodas, energy drinks, and candy bars would no longer be paid for by taxpayers. Very quickly this exemption (just like alcohol & tobacco which are now exempt from EBT payments) would change consumer behavior and over time, and would in turn make a huge improvement in our nation's health! If anyone agrees with this common sense solution, please let your local politicians know. If enough people speak up, maybe someday we can make this a reality.

ACTION ITEM 1.0

If you feel inclined to write a letter or send an e-mail to your local government official about a junk food tax, that's great. However, there's a quicker, easier action you can take today, that will only take 2 to 3 minutes. Go to www.Change.org, www.thepetitionsite.com, (or any other petition website) and search for any common sense food or healthcare petition. In the form, simply type your name and e-mail address. These petition companies will not ask your age, background, marriage status, phone number or any other personal information. Most on-line petitions are very simple to fill out (usually in a just a few seconds) and perhaps you can help make a difference!

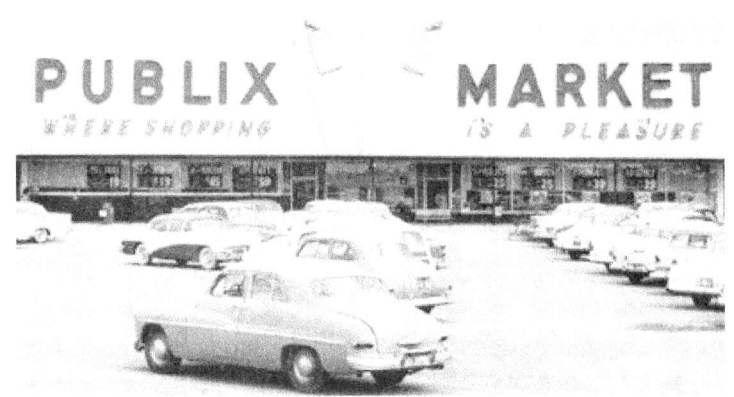

Just a few decades ago, Publix (a Southeastern U.S. super market chain) was actually called a Super 'Market'.

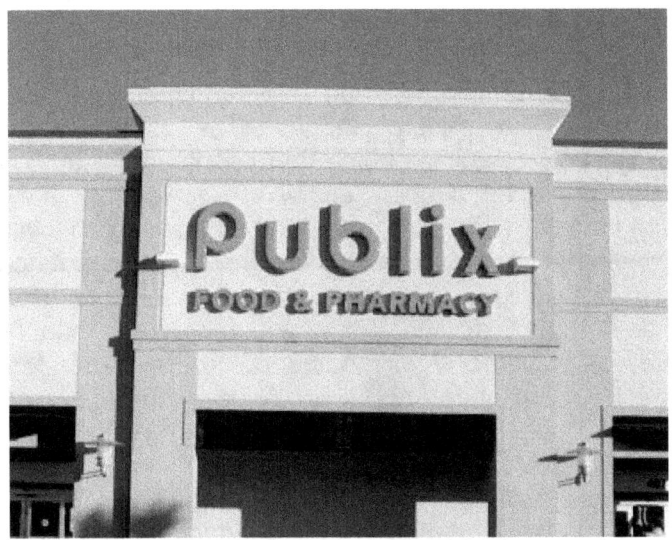

The new slogan for Publix: 'Food & Pharmacy' since a large portion of their business is now from prescription drugs.

Chapter 2.
How BAD is the Food You're Eating Today?

It still pains me when I'm in line at the grocery store to see people in the check out line loaded up with boxes, packages, containers, cans and shrink wrapped foods that have been processed, refined, salted, fortified, preserved, treated or laden with sugar or HFCS (high fructose corn syrup). My cart usually contains vegetables, sprouts, fruits, nuts and often a can or two of black (or kidney) beans. It's estimated in today's grocery stores at least 80% of all grocery products are sugar laden, highly processed, packaged foods while only 10 to 20% are *real* foods that grow out of the ground or hang on a tree, bush or vine. It's an eye-opening experience if you ever discover the marketing schemes, shelf placement and labeling strategies that sell billions in groceries every year. For several years in my seminars, I've shown slides of 20 different food products from a grocery store and challenge the audience to find at least one food item that is all-natural and completely healthy. The packaging and labeling is often so misleading that people in the audience usually cannot tell what's healthy anymore! Now, I'm not saying that 100% of your food should be real (especially if you're going on a two-week camping trip and you can't take all live perishable foods), but if you want to be healthy and have the vitality and energy you deserve, at least 80% (preferably more) of your foods should be real, live foods! In the following chapters, I'll break down the specifics of different foods including all these different processed, refined foods, meats, poultry, fish, frozen foods, etc. and answer some of the questions that arise from all these different foods. I'll also look at the big dairy myth as well as point out the realities of the beverage industry including so-called 'healthy' water, teas, fruit juices, etc. In the mean time, there are some positive changes going on in certain communities. We're starting to see more organic foods offered as well as more farmers markets popping up around the country as more people are being educated about eating real, healthy foods. In different cities, communities are banding together to grow their own real food in community gardens. This not only saves people money on their grocery bill, but provides healthy foods while educating children about natural foods instead of the pizza, hot dogs, chicken nuggets, french fries, etc. still served in many public schools. Apartment dwellers with limited space are starting to grow their own vegetables with hydroponic systems, which is also exciting. For anyone who doesn't live close to a grocery store or market with healthy real food offerings, or for others who simply can't seem to find to find the time to grocery shop, there are several new websites and services to help get real, healthy foods from the farm right to your table with a few clicks of your mouse or via your smartphone. Visit www.FarmtoPeople.com or www.InstaCart.com. As demand increases, you'll find more services like this expanding to cities all over the country.

ACTION ITEM 2.0
Make a commitment to purchase at least one extra real food this week; preferably not a frozen food. Purchase a real vegetable, fruit, legume, bag of nuts, etc. Make sure that this food grows out of the ground or hangs from a tree. If you can't afford organic that's OK, but make sure you get *some* real food (or more real food) this week to benefit your health! This habit will grow on you until one day you're eating mostly real food!

Chapter 3.
'Quick & Easy'

Often in our fast paced lives we don't always have time for nutritious, healthy meals. Sometimes when you're running late for work and don't have time to cook up a large breakfast (the most important meal of the day), you might stop by Starbucks for a coffee and muffin, or zip through the drive-through at McDonald's and order 'Breakfast Combo # 3' (whatever that is?). Another scenario is you're driving cross-country on a road trip and there simply aren't that many healthy food choices available and/or open late at night. The reliable go-to places: the gas station store, mini-mart, or the typical fast food places are more likely to be open around the clock. There are always challenges when traveling, but I'm going to plant the seed here for some healthy options. My older brother (Peter) faced a big challenge a few years ago (before he turned his health around) as he has an extremely busy travel schedule. Sometimes Peter travels three weeks out of the month and most of his travel is throughout Asia. He would mention to me that he might have a layover in Tokyo for a few hours before heading on to Manila, or back to his home in Bangkok and often times his layovers or stops would be late at night when many of the airport restaurants and shops were closed. Sometimes the only late night options available at these airports are vending machines, fast food, or a 24-hour coffee shop. Certainly not many healthy food options. With all of these quick and easy (fast food) options, the problem should be obvious - the food is not fresh and it's usually processed with added chemicals and preservatives. The double whammy is that many of these foods are microwaved (zapped with radioactive energy). There are several problems with eating microwaved food on a regular basis, and Lizette Borreli (a writer for Medical Daily) shares five of the big ones [3-1]: 1) Microwaves zap food nutrition: the dielectric heating of microwaves can destroy or deplete the nutritional value of the original food. 2) Microwaves destroy breast milk and vitamin B-12: in a study published in the Journal of Agricultural and Food Chemistry, researchers decided to examine the effects of microwave heating on the loss of vitamin B-12 in foods like raw beef, pork, and milk. The results of the study show there was a 30 to 40% loss of the vitamins when the foods received microwave exposure. The powerful bacteria-fighting agents in breast milk are also destroyed by microwave heating.   3) Microwaves can create carcinogens in food: the assembling or packaging of microwavable foods are found to contain toxic chemicals such as BPA, polyethylene terpthalate (PET), benzene, toluene, and xylene says www.Foodbabe.com. The plastic containers used to heat these microwave meals have been found to release the carcinogens along with other harmful toxins into your food, which can then be absorbed by your body.   4) Microwaves can change the makeup of your blood: in a Swiss clinical study, researchers found that blood actually changes in individuals who consumed microwaved milk and vegetables. The eight participants in the study ate a series of food prepared in different ways, including food heated in the microwave. The results of the study showed red blood cells decreased while white cell levels increased, along with cholesterol levels.   5) Microwaves can change your heart rate: microwaves can produce effects on your body instantly due to the 2.4 GHz radiation - the frequency of radiation emitted by microwave ovens. A study conducted by Dr. Magda Havas of Trent University found the levels of radiation emitted by a microwave affect both heart rate and heart rate variability. These levels are within federal safety guidelines, but tend to cause immediate and dramatic changes in heart rate. The study warns people: "If you experience irregular heart beat or any chest pain and regularly eat microwaved food, it might be best to discontinue use". Now, I'm NOT trying to get anyone to stop eating fast foods or throw their microwave ovens out, but these facts might be worth considering how much microwave food you eat on a regular basis. Food for thought? Getting back to the challenge of eating healthy, many years ago I was a traveling sales representative for Xerox Corporation (often eating lunch and dinner in my car), and I'd tell myself all sorts of lame excuses: "I'm way too busy", "I'm on the road all day", "I just can't find the time for a healthy meal". The reality is I was uneducated about different healthy options and would often justify to myself why a Wendy's combo meal was the only option late at night while traveling on the road. So what's the solution? Two Tips: 1) plan ahead, and

2) substitute options! Let me give you two real world examples this past week. I was working on a guerilla-style film shoot last week on the streets of Century City. We had no craft service set up, no catering company, so we were on our own filming a project with a small crew working from 8:00 am until 5:00 pm with a 15-minute pizza break for lunch. Knowing this, I planned ahead - I had a large, nutritious breakfast at home (a vegetable-fruit smoothie with kale, carrots, banana & avocado) and also packed home made trail mix for a snack. I drank tons of water all day since we were out in the hot sun, and when lunch came I substituted a salad from a local restaurant instead of the free pepperoni pizza provided for us. Another great nutrition tip (when traveling or working long hours - especially the potential 14 or 15 hour film shoots) is I always bring a small 'Green Drink' sleeve packet (see photo below) that you can get at any Sprouts or Whole Foods store. A small packet will fit in your pocket and provide you two complete healthy green drinks during the day. Just pour ½ a packet into your large bottled water, shake and voila... you' re drinking pure alkaline, energizing plant food! (I'll explain more about alkalizing and energizing in a future chapter). If you also need a little 'pick me up', some of the green drinks have green tea as one of their many ingredients, so you'll get a small amount caffeine in a healthier form than drinking coffee or cola. Another real world example was a 12-mile day hike I went on last month with friends in the San Gabriel mountains. We all met up at a gas station convenience store in the small town of Azuza. This was the last place to get any food or supplies before we drove another 20 minutes to the base of the mountain to start our hike. Once again, I had a large vegetable-fruit smoothie as my breakfast at home. I also packed two bananas, a large bag of trail mix, three large bottled waters, and a full sleeve of the green drink I mentioned above. A few of my fellow hikers stumbled into the convenience store to get their morning coffees and energy drinks, beef jerky, over priced granola bars, Gatorade, PowerAde, water, etc. My bananas and trail mix were not only all natural, but by planning ahead I didn't waste $10.00 at that convenience store or have any temptations to make poor food choices while out on the trail. (I'll discuss the many problems you may not be aware of with energy bars and sports drinks in

a later chapter). In addition to choosing healthy snacks, my final tip to anyone I coach is to drink lots of water. Water is the most important element your body needs, more than anything else on the planet. Since your body is made up of 60 to 70% water, and the earth is comprised of 71% water, it should be common sense that you need to drink a great deal of water, yet most busy people either forget to hydrate sufficiently, or they're drinking coffee, energy drinks, sodas, or flavored waters, etc. which all actually dehydrate you! Water (and nothing else) is what you need to drink the most of. Not only will you get an energy boost from keeping super hydrated, but when filling up with water during the day, you tend to not be quite as hungry for food, which will help fight the urge for unhealthy snacks while traveling or in between your main meals.

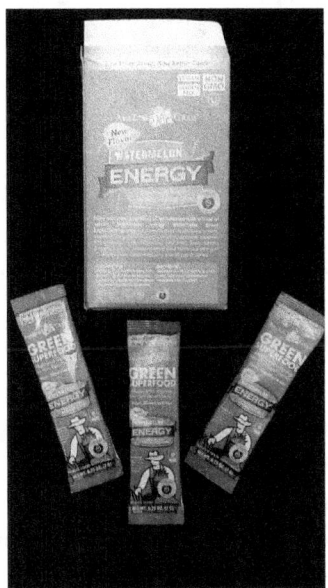

My 'Quick & Easy' healthy snack drink!

Here's an important story I'd like to share about the long term effects of keeping your habit of grabbing quick and easy foods if you're doing this on a regular basis. I attended a focus group several years in Los Angeles on fast foods and one incident still haunts me to this day. One of the large fast food chains paid us each $100.00 for an hour of our time to find out our perception of fast foods and eating habits. The focus group moderator went around the room asking questions until she stopped at this one poor lady. This lady (Ellen) had been laid off her job and her husband didn't make much money to begin with. He was only able to find part time work and they had 3 kids to feed. Ellen described in detail how she would drive her kids to school every day and on the way she would order four Wendy's Jr. bacon cheeseburgers for 99 cents each and four sodas. She would cut each of these bacon cheeseburgers in half, so each child would get a meal for less than 50 cents each. The entire focus group had admitted earlier to seeing the documentaries "Food Inc." and "Super Size Me", so needless to say when we listened to this poor, embarrassed lady describe how she'd been feeding her children for the past two years (every single day), we were flabbergasted. Nobody commented and the room fell silent while we listened to Ellen's story. Ellen sensing from the group that this was wrong, literally broke down in tears crying: "I know this is so wrong what I'm doing to my kids. And I know it is not good for them as they often get sick, but I don't know what else I can possibly do to feed them when they are screaming that they are always hungry...".

Inside I was crying for this lady and for her kids whom I had never met. Now this true story may be a little extreme, but is it any wonder why her kids are often sick if every single day if she's feeding them fast food loaded with toxins? You may remember Morgan Spurlock (the director and star of "Super Size Me") who started vomiting in the McDonald's parking lot after a few days of his 'McDonald's only' diet! If you put a consistent stream of toxins and poisons into our bodies each day, you will get sick, you will probably develop an illness or disease, and you may likely get cancer and die! Decide to do the Action Item below and over time this decision will change your health and your life!

ACTION ITEM 3.0

Grab a pen and paper and write out one of the snacks you eat on a daily basis, which you know are probably unhealthy (ex. potato chips, cookies, donuts, candy bar, etc.). Take your pen and put a big 'X' through one of those snacks and decide to replace that unhealthy snack with a natural, healthy choice. (ex. an apple, banana, carrots, trail mix, etc.). Congratulations, this 60-second action item you just chose will start to make a positive difference in your health!

Chapter 4.
GMOs

GMOs (Genetically Modified Organisms) are animal, plant, or microorganisms that have been significantly altered either by selectively cross-breeding or genetically altered engineering. While many concerns have been raised about GMOs the last few years, I can't say with 100% certainty if GMOs are harmful to one's health, because for starters I haven't been able to go on a long term diet (for at least 30 days) with absolute certainty that none of my food was genetically altered and there simply hasn't been enough conclusive evidence. There have also been a few conflicting studies. However, my concern is that I've read multiple studies revealing much of the U.S. staple crops (like corn) are now genetically engineered to either be herbicide resistant (Roundup ready) or produce it's own insecticide (Bt Toxin). Since insects have become more resistant to these powerful herbicides and poisons, the farmers have been using stronger and higher quantities of pesticides. This raises some health questions if we're eating large amounts of this food. Could this possibly be leading to the higher prevalence in food allergies, sickness, disease and cancer we now see? My hope is that there will be more thorough testing of GMOs in the coming years. My other concern about GMOs are the politics involved since a few countries have banned GMOs outright. There are also several countries that have allowed GMOs with the simple caveat that all food products be labeled (GMO or non-GMO) and there is a reason for this. Most people simply want to know exactly what's in their food! Friends and clients ask me all the time: "Are GMOs bad for my health and do GMOs cause health problems?" and my response is always the same. "I can't say with certainty, but I do have a few questions and concerns". Almost all of my educated friends feel the same way. In fact, in November of 2012, there was the widely discussed Proposition # 37 - a California statewide ballot measure that would have required labeling of genetically engineered food. I spoke to hundreds of friends, family members, and even strangers in different grocery stores who all thought the simple act of labeling would be a great compromise to at least allow consumers to make a choice. I was shocked that the most widely discussed proposition in years (Proposition # 37) did not pass, as I hadn't met a single registered voter I spoke to who voted against it. Anyway, if you live in a different state that in the future has a similar proposition, I encourage you to at least support labeling the food you buy for you and your family... this is common sense. In the meantime, I sometimes eat GMO food (as it's almost possible to avoid), but when I see this small label below, I make the personal choice to buy non-GMO (all natural) food until all the facts are in.

ACTION ITEM 4.0
The next time you go to the grocery store, start actively looking for the Non-GMO label. Make the decision (if there's not a huge price differential) to buy Non-GMO food. It's better for the environment and it will give you some peace of mind!

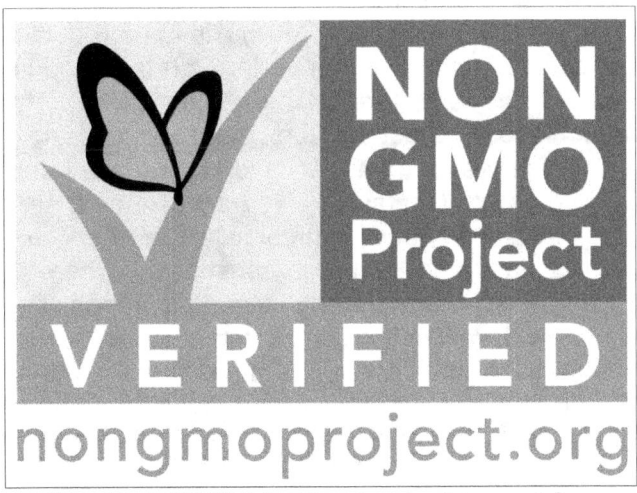

The Non-GMO label to start looking out for.

Chapter 5.
'Factory Farmed' Meats

I always disclose that I'm not a vegetarian, so it would be hypocritical of me to advise you or anybody else not to eat meat. However, several years ago I changed my lifestyle where I don't buy any meat to prepare at home and generally don't order meat (or meat products) when I'm at a restaurant. If I'm out with friends or family or attending a special event where they happen to serve meat, I will occasionally have and enjoy meat. Since drastically reducing my intake of meat and consuming a mostly plant-based diet, I've never felt better. Americans eat more meat per capita (including pork, poultry, and beef) than any country in the world, more than 175 lbs. per person, per year. [5-1] That number, which includes lots of cheap meats, seems to be increasing every year. It's estimated in the United States that 90% of all the meat consumed today comes from factory farms. Essentially these are massive industrialized farm operations in which large numbers of livestock (often thousands) are raised indoors under one roof in conditions intended to maximize production at minimal cost. Whether it's a drive-through fast food joint, a restaurant, a grocery store or the freezer section of a big box super store, most of the meat (unless specially labeled) is the less expensive variety and usually not all-natural or organic. The last five years working on set of all the films, TV shows, and commercials I've been on, I did an informal study and kept a spreadsheet of where all the meat came from the different catering companies. After every lunch, I'd walk to the back of the catering tent or food truck (where the chefs were) to thank them for the meal. Out of 200 informal interviews I did over 5 years, 181 of the meals were confirmed NOT to have organic meats. [5-2] That means that over 90% of the meals served were factory farmed meats. The few times that all-natural, open range, organic meats were served, the catering company displayed signs bragging about the special meal and sometimes, special menus were printed up. I certainly do not blame the studios, networks, or the producers at all, since our meals are provided for free and the employers of each show have to feed between 100 to 200 people each day when you add up all the cast, crew, background talent, vendors, etc. working on a single day. Plus the entire crew has to be fed quickly before returning back to work. Managing costs is a standard and responsible business practice. If you' re 100% honest with yourself (as I was with my study on film & TV sets, and when I inquired about my mother's meat purchasing habits at home), you need to take a hard look at where your meat comes from and how much you paid for it. Naturally raised, organic meat costs *at least* two to three times more than regular meat! For example: you can find chicken meat priced around $2.00 per lb., but if you want meat from chickens that have been raised outside of cages and able to walk around, allowed to see daylight, that have been fed healthy, organic (non-GMO) feed, and not given any antibiotics, this will usually cost you more than double (on average $4.00 to $6.00 per lb.). It's the same scenario for beef. If you're 100% truthful about the burgers or steaks you and your family eat on a regular basis, there are obvious reasons why all-natural, organically raised, grass-fed beef costs 250% to 400% more than the majority of beef products on sale at your grocery store. In addition to cheap, GMO feed given to most cattle, they are often given antibiotics along with steroids and growth hormones which greatly help accelerate the maturation of a cow from birth to slaughter. In the mid 1900's the maturity rate of a steer was 5 years while in 2013 the maturity rate of a steer was only 15 months! [5-3] There is enormous pressure on the meat conglomerates to keep shortening that maturity rate from fast food restaurants and big box stores like Wal-Mart where consumers expect to find low prices for the burgers they feed their families. There are a multitude of different beef products and cuts, but the average ground beef that costs $2.00 per lb. can easily run about $5.00 to $6.00 per lb. for the healthiest, all-natural, organic option. For most families on a tight budget, this is a considerable price difference to pay every week at the grocery store when trying to make ends meet. Anyone who went to a fast food restaurant in the mid-1980's remembers the $0.99 burger or when the $1.00 value meal 'price wars' started between the big chains like McDonald's, Wendy's, Burger King, etc. What shocks most economists is that this same $1.00 price war has been going on now for 30 years as most fast food restaurants still have a burger offering for just one dollar! Can you name a single product after 30 years of inflation and price increases that has stayed the same exact price? I can't, but as mentioned above the chemists, scientists, and breeders have figured out a way to grow cattle, chickens, and pigs faster and cheaper than ever before. There are moral and ethical issues about factory farming and there are serious environmental hazards and issues about widespread factory farming which especially impact people living near these massive complexes where thousands of these animals are raised. (This book is not going to delve into those issues; I'll let you do your own research if you are interested). My focus here is to discuss the possible health issues of eating factory-farmed meat. For those of you who have the financial means to buy all-natural, organically raised meat, I applaud you. I also want to point out that more and more medical doctors and even retired heart surgeons like Dr. Caldwell Esselstyn (who served as President of Staff at the legendary Cleveland Clinic) are raising concerns about eating too much meat (especially red meat) and the effect it may have on heart disease. Over the years, Dr. Esselstyn has published over 150 medical studies concluding that people who consumed meat were much more likely to have high cholesterol, elevated blood pressure, and heart disease than people on a plant-based diet. According to the CDC (Centers for Disease Control and Prevention), about 610,000 Americans die from heart disease each year... that's 1 in every 4 deaths! [5-4] If you want to know all the facts about carnivorous diets (like in the U.S. where we eat more meat per person than almost any other country in the world), I suggest you and your loved ones watch the documentary film: "Forks Over Knives" where many medical doctors, cardiac experts, and nutritionists reveal startling facts, as well as show you how easy it is to reverse most medical conditions and even heart disease! The key is you have to be willing to make some changes in your diet. The most incredible experiment (which will never happen again in history) proves the negative effect that meat (and dairy) can have on an entire population, occurred during World War II in Norway. There are numerous historical studies that show that heart disease between 1940 and 1945 dropped by over 50%! In 1940 when Hitler and the Nazi regime occupied Norway, one of the first things the Nazis did was to confiscate all local livestock. The meat, cheese, milk, and eggs were to provide sustenance for the German soldiers and officers. During that short time when the entire Norwegian population (for the most part) ate vegetarian, you can see in the graph below what happened! Shortly following the end of the war in 1945, the circulatory diseases started ticking up again when the Norwegians started regaining their livestock and started eating meat and dairy products again. One last bit of information which I've been telling my clients for years (and I was finally vindicated last year when many mainstream media and reports revealed the truth about red and processed meats): "The World Health Organization has classified processed meats - including ham, salami, sausages and hot dogs as a Class 1 carcinogen, which means that there is strong evidence that processed meats cause cancer. Red meat (such as beef, lamb and pork) has been classified as a probable cause of cancer. [5-5] The reasoning behind this is that there are often all sorts of preservatives, additives, curing, smoking added to processed meats. The science behind red meat not being healthy for anyone to eat every day is the fact that red meat contains uric acid. With a western diet, that is already highly acidic, adding more acid and additional cholesterol from red meat is not the healthiest choice. As part of my daily research yesterday, I was listening to a radio interview of Dr. David Katz who is the Founding Director of Yale University Prevention Research Center and President of the American College of Lifestyle Medicine - to name a few of his accomplishments. The important summary of his interview came down to three simple words. His unequivocal advice (with all his years of research) was no matter whether you eat red meat once a day, once a week or twice a month, his powerful take-away that he repeated at least five times was: "Eat less red meat." Please do your own research and no matter what the National Cattlemen's Beef Association, or American Association of Meat Processors claim, there are some health risks of eating meat (especially red meat) every day. I'm not suggesting that you stop eating all meat, however I strongly urge my family members, loved ones and my clients to scale back the amount of meat they consume for their own health benefits. For those who choose to go vegetarian or vegan, I applaud you even more and you'll see many real world examples of healthy vegetarians in chapter 13.

ACTION ITEM 5.0
Get 100% honest with yourself about the meats you may be eating. Are you spending 2 to 3 times more money to buy all-natural, organic meats? Are you eating red meat or processed meat (bacon, salami, pepperoni, etc.) 3 times per week or more? Set a new goal to eat less meat and substitute a few plant based meals or fish. This simple action item will be one more step towards better health!

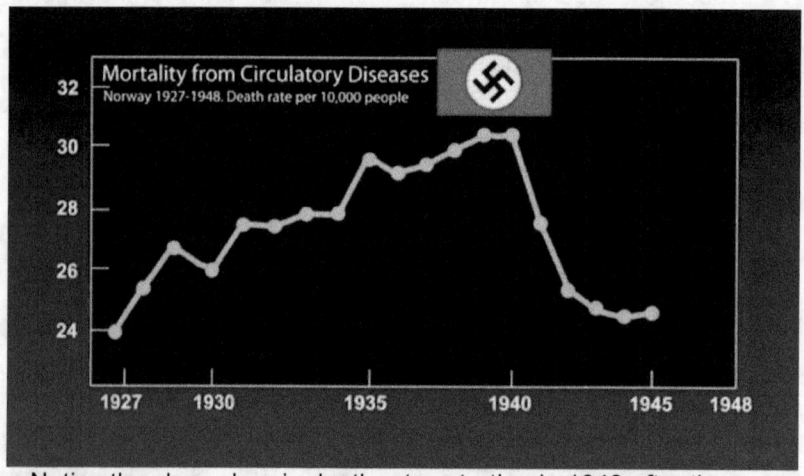

Notice the sharp drop in death rates starting in 1940 after the Nazi's put the entire Norwegian population on a plant-based diet.

Chapter 6.
Poultry...Fowl or Foul?

I could share many pages of statistics of how 'foul' most chicken meat in the U.S. is with the growing amounts of antibiotics pumped into the sick birds. A record of nearly 29.9 billion pounds of drugs was pumped into livestock in 2011 according to www.MotherJones.com.[6-1] Many of these birds are so sick that every day inside the factory farms, dozens of chickens (often many more) are found dead on the feces covered, dark floors of the massive hen houses. In 1957 the average growth period for a broiler chicken to reach slaughter weight was 63 days. By the 1990's the number of growth days had been reduced to 38 and the amount of feed required halved! [6-2] With the help of lots of antibiotics and GMO feed, the scientists employed by the large chicken conglomerates keep shrinking the growth cycle while containing the costs of raising the birds. This is the magic of how the fast food companies have been able to keep the prices of their chicken sandwiches and nuggets down so low vs. the annual inflation rates of most other products. Now the truly organic chickens (fed 100% organic food, grown with no pesticides, fed zero antibiotics, and are given free range access to the outdoors and sunlight) are considered one of the healthiest meats. But, the reality is that all-natural, organic chicken meat can cost $4.00 to $6.00 per lb. or more! The majority of the chicken meat in the U.S. is factory farmed and found in fast foods, most restaurants, and the packages most people buy at their local grocery stores cost between $1.50 to $2.50 per lb.

I used to look at chicken as the healthier meat alternative and always ate chicken (rather than beef, pork, or lamb) when working on film or TV sets four or five days every week. I also used to believe that to remain strong and healthy I needed animal protein, so I'd add chicken meat into my vegetable soup or salad - which I ate most days for lunch when working at home. As mentioned in the previous chapter, I discovered to my horror that over 90% of all the film & TV show catering companies were not serving us organic chicken. Once again, I don't blame them, or the production companies when they're serving complimentary lunches to over 100 cast, crew, extra, and vendors every day while on tight budgets. However, I gave myself a reality check about the food I was eating every day and asked myself if I wanted to continue the same route or make a shift towards better health. So about five years ago, I decided to get honest with myself about the chicken I was eating. There was no way that eating that much cheap chicken was good for me, so I quit cold turkey! I decided to go vegetarian or eat fish the days I would be working on set. I also cut out all chicken from my soups and/or salads at home. I now substitute some spinach, kale, sprouts, mushrooms, beans, and/or lentils - which are all better sources of protein. Within a few weeks, I noticed I felt better after eating! I had more energy, was less bloated, and also felt proud about contributing less to the factory farm machines, since as a consumer I stopped buying chicken meat at home. My clients who also stopped eating chicken (or at least the cheap chicken) noticed that they also felt better. I firmly believe that eating less cheap chicken and other meats has been one of the factors that helped many of my clients get off their prescription drugs. As mentioned, just because I went 'cold turkey' and stopped eating cheap chicken several days a week, doesn't mean I don't enjoy a chicken breast or wing now and then, but I'm no longer kidding myself that all chicken is the healthiest meat. Some fowl simply needs to be called 'foul'!

ACTION ITEM 6.0

Find out exactly where the poultry you eat is coming from. Make a decision today to start buying organic on occasion and cut or reduce the cheap, factory farmed chicken out of your diet.

Chapter 7.
If it Sounds 'Fishy', It Usually Is!

As mentioned, about 5 years ago I switched my most common source of animal protein from chicken to fish and vegetables, once I realized that every film and TV show I worked on was purchasing the lower priced chicken. In the previous chapter on poultry, you just read about the massive amount of antibiotics given to healthy chickens, turkeys, etc. to make the fowl grow much faster and also to prevent sickness from spreading in the cramped, dark, factory-farm living conditions. It's no secret that in the past 20 years, antibiotics have become much less effective in their ability to treat us, and in addition to the additional prescriptions doctors are writing for their patients, I believe the primary reason is the massive amount of antibiotics in our factory farmed animals (especially in America's most popular meat - chicken). In 2010, the United States used over 29 million pounds of antibiotics in livestock per year [7-1].The amount of antibiotics used has increased in the U.S. and will exponentially increase in other countries like China with their brand new insatiable appetite for meat. While TIME Magazine reported that "80% of antibiotics sold in the U.S. are used on mostly healthy animals on factory farms" [7-2], a recent report by the Union of Concerned Scientists found that nearly 90% of the total use of antimicrobials in the United States was for non-therapeutic purposes in agricultural production. These statistics are shocking! The World Health Organization has now classified the emergence of antibiotic-resistant bacteria as a global crisis. In the U.S., these 'superbugs' sicken more than 2 million people a year. Of those, 23,000 people die according to the CDC. [7-3] Knowing what I'd discovered after a good year or so of research, I decided to eat more fish when it was offered on set instead of chicken. My favorite fish to eat when offered is salmon. I limit my intake of bigger open water fish like tuna and swordfish due to the increasing mercury levels. Not to digress here too much, but in case you were not aware, eating too much sushi or any kind of larger fish (higher up the food chain) can be very dangerous with the increased mercury levels currently found in these fish, and of course the possible radiation from the partial meltdown of the Fukushima, Japan nuclear power plant. The best personal example I can share is the well-known Hollywood actress - Daphne Zuniga who suffered from severe mercury poisoning who had at times, been eating sushi four times per week. At one point, Daphne became so sick that she was taken to the emergency room and had to take some time off from acting. Her symptoms included weakness, headaches, skin rashes, etc. Daphne stopped consuming fish altogether and when I met her at a charity event in 2014, she was back in great health and looked amazing! I applaud Daphne for bringing awareness to this mercury problem in fish and all the great charity work she now does for different projects including the Los Angeles River Revitalization Corporation. I don't want to scare you from never eating large game fish again like tuna, swordfish, cod, etc. on occasion. However if you eat a lot of these larger types of saltwater fish, I encourage you to do your own research on this mercury issue. Getting back to the real 'fishy' story I uncovered most recently was about factory-farmed fish. After finding out the massive amounts of antibiotics the big chicken conglomerates were pumping into the chicken I was eating on set made me queasy, I started substituting fish. The good news is that fish is offered as an option on the film and TV show catering trucks almost every day. Before I started my in depth research, I noticed there was a big shift away from tuna, swordfish, and salmon to more tilapia. It seemed like almost every single day (no exaggeration) the 'fish of the day' was tilapia (or a similar white fish), so I started inquiring why? As mentioned earlier, when you're feeding hundreds of people, cost is an issue and in many cases this new, favored and increasing popular catch of the day (tilapia), is very inexpensive - often running between $1.00 to $2.00 per lb. It's also one of the most popular fish to raise in fish farms (or fish factories) over in Vietnam, Thailand and China. So even with the long, expensive shipping costs all the way around the world from Asia to the United States and eventually on to our dinner plate, how was this tilapia still so much cheaper than all the other fish in the grocery store? After all, they've been farming salmon for many years up in the Pacific Northwest (which I saw first hand off of Orcas Island, WA) and it is not a pretty sight. I wondered why it was so much more expensive (even without the shipping costs) than the factory farmed raised tilapia on the other side of the world? Since there's no equivalent agency like the FDA (Food & Drug Administration) in these Asian countries and China' s own government has admitted they don't have the best oversight over food production in the country, profit often comes before food safety. To make matters worse, the minimal oversight and regulations China does have can't possibly check or catch all of the business operations there. First and foremost, those fish farms are trying to maximize profits and happen to be in the most populated country in the world. In addition to raising food to feed 1.4 billion people, China has found it profitable to export to over 100 other countries around the world including the United States where their factory farmed fish end up at your local grocery store. Just as there is an acceptable death rate in the chicken factory farms, there is an acceptable death rate on these large fish farms. If a certain percentage of fish in their small, overcrowded pens die and with their bloated stomachs end up floating around with the thousands of other fish, that' s OK, so long as the farmers can still get enough fish to market. Just like the chicken problem, it's common to feed antibiotics to the young fish to make them grow faster and so they have a better chance of surviving the horrid living conditions in the over crowded pens. Economics 101: keep your inputs (cost) of the product as low as possible and sell at the highest price point to yield the highest profit. When I drove by the salmon factory farm off of Orcas Island, I could see the crowded pens of fish and caught a whiff of their stink (mostly fish excrement) where the thousands of fish had been penned up for a long time. If you were to visit an Asian factory fish farm, you might well see the filth and the many dead fish bobbing on the surface of the water. According to many investigations including a recent piece by Business Insider: "Tilapia in China's fish farms, are fed pig and goose manure - even though it contains salmonella and makes the tilapia more susceptible to disease". [7-4] Once again, the farmers who are out to make a profit are doing whatever they can to lower the costs of the product, regardless if some of the fish die along the way. In countless other journalistic investigations it's revealed that in addition to GMO corn and soy (cheap feed), it's common for farmed fish to be fed antibiotics, chemicals, ground up chicken parts and raw sewage to fatten them up. An ABC News piece tries to put the American public at ease by explaining: "The FDA states there is no imminent threat to the public health, because of the low levels of contaminants. But the banned substances could cause serious health problems if consumed over a long period of time". Once again, don't just take my word for it. Ask yourself why is some fish priced 250 to 400% higher than other fish in the same fish section at your grocery store? My guess is that it's factory farm raised in China or some other Asian country. My suggestion is to look at the bottom left hand corner of the package and you'll see in very fine print (normally 10 font or smaller): "Farmed in China". When you read that label, you might think twice about what you want to feed your loved ones at home. As the old saying goes, "If it sounds fishy, it usually is"!

ACTION ITEM 7.0
The next time you shop for fish, take a close look at the bottom left hand corner of the package to check if it was farm raised, and if so in what country? Printed on the clear plastic wrap in a tiny 9 or 10 font, it will read: "Farm raised in _____ (name of the country)". Take charge of the fish you're eating and make a healthier decision.

Chapter 8.
The Dairy Myth

Almost ten years ago, I was hired by Calpers to do Medco® presentations to thousands of retired teachers and public school employees around California. I noticed a plethora of flyers, pamphlets and posters at every school promoting the "Calcium Connection... food and activity choices that help you build and keep strong bones". The campaign promoted milk, milk products, yogurt, cheese, etc. and was sponsored by the Dairy Council of California. You might remember the 'Food Pyramid' introduced by the USDA (United States Department of Agriculture) decades ago? This pyramid put dairy products at the top of the food chain and recommended 2 to 3 servings every day. The famous 'Got Milk?' advertising campaign that encouraged the consumption of cow's milk was created for the California Milk Processor Board in 1993, and later was licensed for use by milk processors and dairy farmers. You should always pay attention to who is behind the message promoting any type of food industry. I'm not saying never drink cow's milk, but I'm not sure 2 to 3 dairy servings every day is ideal for your health anymore. In observational studies, higher dairy intake has been linked to increased risk of several different cancers, higher rates of multiple sclerosis, has been shown to promote increased cholesterol levels and atherosclerosis, has been found to be pro-inflammatory and actually is linked to models of aging. Higher milk intake has been linked to acne, constipation and ear infections. Milk is perhaps the most common self-reported food allergen in the world with much of the world's population unable to adequately digest milk due to lactose intolerance.[8-1] The most disturbing news is in many cases dairy (including milk) can cause calcium loss. There are dozens of studies and reports supporting this fact, so I'll let you do your own research, but here's a summary below about how milk became a profitable, mainstream 'cash cow'. One of the first radical changes to our food began in the late 1800's after Louis Pasteur invented the pasteurization process in France. One of the first products in the U.S. to be pasteurized was milk by being exposed briefly to high (often scalding) temperatures to destroy and kill microorganisms and prevent fermentation. There is often a debate about drinking pasteurized and homogenized milk as opposed to drinking raw milk coming from a small farm, grass raised dairy cow. There were (and still are) benefits from pasteurization, but it's odd that humans are the only animals on the planet who: 1) drink milk from a completely different animal species and 2) keep drinking milk our entire lives after the weaning period. Now with the massive increase in dairy consumption (including milk, cream, cheese, yogurt, ice cream, etc.) there have been literally thousands of studies proving that dairy foods can create all kinds of health problems from a minor food allergy to serious problems like heart disease, arthritis, and osteoporosis. This last one stuns people, but here's the truth... a 12-year Harvard study of 80,000 nurses showed that a high intake of commercial milk appeared to actually increase the risk of bone fractures! Higher milk consumption (with all that great calcium medical doctors and the American Dairy Association tell us to drink every day) actually leads to higher rates of osteoporosis! [8-2] There are two reasons for this: first, when milk is pasteurized and homogenized, your body can't absorb or use all the calcium. Second, modern day milk contains animal proteins and acids which actually cause the body to leach calcium right out of the bones, but more on that in the chapter on acidity later in the book. You read that correctly... the most surprising link is that not only do we barely absorb the calcium in cow's milk (especially if pasteurized), but to make matters worse it actually increases calcium loss from the bones. What an irony this is! Here's how it happens. Like all animal protein, milk helps acidifies the body's pH, which in turn triggers a biological correction. You see, calcium is an excellent acid neutralizer and the biggest storage of calcium in the body is - you guessed it... in the bones. So the very same calcium that our bones need to stay strong is utilized to neutralize the acidifying effect of milk. Once calcium is pulled out of the bones, it leaves the body via the urine, so that the surprising net result after this is an actual calcium deficit. The U.S. has among the highest daily consumption of dairy products in the world and coincidentally we lead other developed nations in osteoporosis, osteopenia and bone density loss! One half (50%) of women in this country over 50 will fracture a bone because of osteoporosis! [8-3] According to another 12 year Harvard Medical study on 77,761 women: "Those who consumed the most calcium from dairy foods broke more bones than those who rarely drank milk." According to the all-encompassing China Study, it concluded: "70% of fracture rate was attributed to consumption of animal protein." [8-4] and "In Nigeria with only a 10% animal - plant protein ratio, fracture rate incidence is 99% lower!" [8-5] Luckily the truth is getting out to the public, and people are switching in droves to plant-based milks including almond, rice and soy milk (which all have plenty of calcium and protein). These milk products are not acidic and are also more readily absorbable by the human body. You may have noticed this expanded plant-based milk selection (as well as dairy free yogurts and cheeses) in your local grocery and health food stores. I don't think that drinking a small glass of cow's milk on occasion will hurt you, but I must confess, I myself and most of my friends I speak with about this don't drink traditional milk anymore. This whole 'Dairy' push might really just be a myth. Look carefully at who's promoting the next dairy advertisement you see and do your own research. You be the judge.

ACTION ITEM 8.0
Do your own research on-line or talk to a certified nutritionist to find out the truth about dairy products. Then the next time you're in your grocery store, try out a carton of a plant-based milk. My favorite is almond milk.

Chapter 9.
**Our 'Acid' Lifestyle is Killing Us,
but a Boon for the Antacid Drug Industry.**

The 'Acid' Lifestyle most people have is a great boon for the antacid industry, but it's also a contributing factor of cancer, sickness, and most diseases! This concept is by far the most important chapter of this book and what has transformed my health the most is the concept of 'alkalizing' my body. To give you an idea how profound proper alkalinity has been to my health, energy and vitality the past few years, I got an A^+ tattooed on my body... and I've never been a tattoo type of guy. My new A^+ tattoo reminds me to "Alkalize + Energize" (eat and drink alkaline, energetic foods) and reinforces how I can always get an incredible, steady supply of alkaline energy (just like an alkaline battery) if I follow the principles I'm laying out for you in this chapter. Understanding the delicate pH balance of your body and the negative effect acid can have is critical to your health. If you read the book Alkalize or Die by Dr. Theodore A. Baroody, you'll understand that managing the pH balance in your body and limiting your acidity levels is a matter of life and death! If you think I'm being dramatic, look around at your family and friends and see if any of them have any life threatening diseases, major illnesses, or cancer? Ask yourself if more people you know are battling arthritis, osteoporosis, gout, or general body aches and pains the past few years? The health epidemic for these ailments in the U.S. is growing out of control, as is obesity. I recently heard that the U.S. was the fattest country in the world and figured the average American citizen was maybe 4 to 5 lbs. heavier than the average citizen from other countries. I was stunned to read the latest weight study revealed by Time Magazine which stated the "average U.S. person weighs in at 180 lbs., outweighing the rest of the world by 43 lbs. per person"! [9-1] My friend Tony Robbins explains very clearly how acid can destroy your body starting at the cellular level with your blood cells. Tony has spent several decades studying, researching, and speaking to the world's top experts in blood, cellular health, energy, and nutrition. Tony's explanation paints a visual picture for you and helps you truly understand alkalinity and encourages you to take action towards perfect health. When several family members and friends died of cancer the last few years, that was a real wake up call for me. After my college roommate and fraternity brother (John Clark) died way too young from cancer, I watched a life changing film called "The Gerson Miracle" which is now available on Netflix as well as on many internet channels. Dr. Max Gerson was a ground breaking German physician who developed The Gerson Therapy (an all-natural alternative dietary therapy), and in 1958 published a book in which he documented curing 50 terminal cancer patients: A Cancer Therapy: Results of 50 Cases. The ground-breaking work Dr. Gerson started is now continued by his daughter Charlotte Gerson who delivers proven results! The success rate The Gerson Clinic has proven is astounding, and you can read direct testimonials from dozens of cancer survivors including people like Susan Morton who share their stories at www.Gerson.org. This legendary clinic now has recovering cancer patients who have survived decades after they were sentenced by Medical Doctors to just a few months left to live! Unfortunately the American Medical Association and the FDA would not let these treatments continue in the U.S., so Charlotte Gerson opened a clinic in Mexico (just south of their San Diego headquarters) and a clinic in Hungary. The whole premise of Dr. Gerson's work and the book Alkalize or Die is that once a body becomes too acidic, it starts breaking down almost everything beginning at the cellular level. Problems may start slowly like fatigue (most Americans can relate to this), allergies, acid reflux, sicknesses (including colds and flu symptoms), disease, and eventually cancer. Another major side effect of a body being too acidic is obesity. The pH scale goes from 0 to 14 with 7 being neutral. Your body's pH should be slightly alkaline at 7.36. Once your body gets lower than 7.36 pH (slightly acidic), all sorts of problems start occurring including obesity. Here's the simple explanation why acidity directly leads to obesity. Your body runs on electricity (starting with your heart which is like an electrical pump) and every part of your body is connected by your nervous system's electric grid. Individual nerve cells (neurons) send signals to other cells as electrochemical waves traveling along thin fibers called axons, so if you stub your toe within a fraction of a second, this information is relayed to your brain which causes you to feel pain and shout "ouch". Now back to the acid problem in our diets and how it can lead to obesity. Your body is extremely sophisticated and has a defense mechanism built in to protect your bones and all of your vital organs. When excess acid is detected (once your ph level gets too far below 7.36), your body's neurons alert the brain: "Hey body... we have too much acid and it looks like there is more acid entering the body... holy crap... danger! We just got an alert that another 64 oz. acidic soda is streaming down the esophagus." What happens next is a survival mechanism: your body starts retaining more and more fat as a buffer to protect your skeletal system, your vital organs, and inner workings of your body from all that excess acid. As Dr. Robert Young explains in his book The pH Miracle, "Obesity is not just created by people eating too much" (although taking in more calories than you burn each day will also lead to becoming overweight), "but by people being too acidic". [9-2] Over 15 years ago when I first started researching the pH balance and this acidity problem, I had an incredible epiphany that I remember to this day. I used to go Bally's Fitness gym on a regular basis (once or twice a week) and there were a few people at the gym who worked out every single day. I noticed one gentleman named Justin in particular who worked out hard-core on the treadmill - often huffing and puffing for a good hour. On certain days Justin would work out different parts of his body including upper body, lower body, medicine balls and even advanced aerobics class for an extreme cardio workout. Other days he would run five miles on the indoor track sprinting the last ¼ mile. Justin bragged about having a good diet and that he didn't drink alcohol or smoke, and he was in his early 30's. Justin was in good overall shape, but for the amount of effort he invested, he should have had a 'six-pack' stomach and a V-shaped torso that you see on professional swimmers or Olympic athletes. Instead Justin had two small 'love handles' on either side of his body just above his hips. I bet that 95% of all the guys over the age of 35 reading this book can relate to those damn love handles that never seem to go away no matter how much they work out. For ladies over 40, there' s the dreaded rear end (butt pad) or the very top back portion of your legs that seem to collect cellulite. Even for people in good shape, it can be maddening to have those extra 4 to 5 lbs. or for some people maybe the extra 10 to 15 lbs. of excess fat in those places that never, ever seem to go away! Well the 'ah-ha' moment for me happened one day after I watched Justin finish a 60 minute treadmill session followed by 30 minutes of core body work out including crunches, sit ups, leg lifts, etc. Justin waved good-bye and seemed proud about completing another intense work out. When he walked through the lobby, he stopped at the vending machine and bought a large bottle of Mountain Dew! Eureka... a light bulb went off in my head that even though Justin said he had a healthy diet and worked out like a maniac 5 to 6 days a week, he was dumping liquid acid (and excess sugar) into his body after his workouts. No wonder Justin could never get rid of his love handles! After more reading, research, and dozens of trials with clients I've worked with, I found the answer to the million dollar question everybody is dying to know: "How can I possibly get rid of my last few lbs. of unwanted fat?" The undisputed answer in all of my research and that we have proven with over 500 clients to date is to eliminate excess acid! A few of my initial clients included actors who needed to lose 10 to 15 lbs. in a 1-week time frame for film roles. I'm not bragging or trying to impress you, but want to impress upon you that most people can lose a significant amount of fat weight (including toxins stored in their bodies) in a very short period of time simply by alkalizing their bodies. Speaking of working out, there's a major trap that many fitness buffs fall into these days which is the new Protein bar craze. Protein bars are a booming business with dozens of brands out now and here's the problem with most of them. They are loaded with way too much protein! If you snack on a protein bar that has 28 to 35 grams of protein, and you eat that bar in one sitting as most people do, that's over twice as much protein as your body can immediately assimilate. The excess protein actually becomes an acid ash. I've even seen well meaning parents send their kids off to school with these mega protein bars and once again, there's no possible way a small kid's body can assimilate that much protein at one time. This whole 'protein hype' is not always healthy, but it's great marketing to sell more protein bars. Once you complete our 7-Day "Alkalize & Energize" cleanse (revealed at the end of this book), the best and most healthy diet (or lifestyle) long term is a balance of protein and carbohydrates with a small amount of fats. Yes... even fat! Another false hype is all these new fat-free foods! This is another ploy to sell more processed food. The reality is a small amount of fat in your diet is not only good for you, but essential to your good health.

You've probably heard about really healthy people including most athletes eating a well balanced diet and also eating 4 (or sometimes 5) smaller meals throughout the day. Instead of overloading your body with one huge meal or a mega-protein bar at one sitting, eating smaller well-balanced meals is easier on your digestive system. This should make more sense to you than eating a huge dinner and lunch or having a late night pig out session in front of the television. I'll cover more on this later on in the book. Ronald Farnham was the contributing author of my first health book: Do These Things or You Will Die and he experimented with us for two (2) years and lost 60 lbs. in his first 90 days simply by alkalizing! 90% of his diet was vegetable juice along with some occasional alkaline, raw vegetables. Ronald's 'before and after' photos are pretty amazing. Without excessive exercise (he did no running, weight lifting, P-90X, etc.), but just by alkalizing his system, the weight fell off Ronald's body like butter. There were several days on his weight loss tracking sheet (very important to have this as well as a target weight goal) that Ronald lost 2 to 3 lbs. per day. I once lost 22 lbs. in 7 days on one of my cleanses! What's really interesting is that every single time (without exception) that Ronald had a strenuous workout like pitching an entire baseball game (Ronald used to be a professional baseball player), his weight loss would stop for 1 or 2 days due to build up of lactic acid! At the end of one of my 7-Day "Alkaline & Energize" cleanses (I religiously start a cleanse every January 1st after the holidays), I decided to keep juicing for one more day, but also decided to lift some weights and also run 4 miles including some wind sprints to the point of muscle fatigue. The next day instead of the scale reading 1 to 2 lbs. less, I was shocked, as I had gained 1.5 lbs! Here is the critical point to learn here... doing strenuous exercise or massive workouts will NOT help you lose weight during this cleanse as you're creating lactic acid in your body. In fact, I tell people during the 7-Day "Alkalize & Energize" cleanse not to do any major exercise! I don't mean to keep beating a dead horse here, but millions of Americans are facing major obesity with the many more having the allergies, sickness, disease, and cancer that often goes along with being acidic and overweight. Too much 'extreme' exercise as well as stress can create more acid in the body which is a bad thing. Another problem of an acidic body is the candida (yeast) which as many as 90% of Americans have in their systems. Candida feed on glucose and this is where the constant sugar cravings come from. The cravings for sugar, sweets, coffee, and in some cases alcohol can be eliminated once you kill off the bulk of candida by alkalizing your system! Don't you want to stop this vicious cycle of overeating, being overweight, and being tired all the time? On the weight issue, be honest with yourself! Whether you're 10 lbs. overweight or 50 lbs. overweight, doing our 7-Day "Alkalize & Energize" cleanse outlined at the end of this book will help you lose weight immediately and give you more energy. If you don't lose weight and you don't feel a vastly improved energy level, simply write us and ask for 100% of your money back! It doesn't matter if you bought this book on Amazon, Kindle, in a bookstore, just send us your purchase receipt along with the book and we'll issue you a 100% refund, no questions asked!

With the massive increase in processed foods with added sugars, salts, artificial flavors, colorings, and preservatives, it's not hard to figure out why most people in the U.S. are not as healthy as the previous generation. Besides the dramatically increased cancer rate (in the past 30 years), here's a great visual to point out how fat we've become in this country. I was once at the famous Griffith Park carousel (you've seen in dozens of movies) which is now fully restored just like it was back in the 1960's. I noticed a sign that read: "Weight limit for riders is 200 lbs." If Disney World posted a sign like that on any of their rides, I'd imagine 25% of all the fathers would not be able to go on the rides with their kids. I know for a fact there are a few ladies out there and some teenage kids who also exceed the 200 lb. weight limit, so they too would not be allowed to have fun on the rides if we upheld the same standards we had just a few decades ago. Getting back to acidity (since excess acid is the root cause of obesity, many diseases, and cancer), I'd like to briefly discuss meat (which contains uric acid) as one of my friend's beliefs about meat are not entirely accurate. One of my friends claimed: "We were born carnivores and we need red meat for protein to stay healthy." Science and history prove something quite different. If you look at early cave men (homo erectus and the earliest forms of homo sapiens), our mutual ancestors were designed to eat mostly organic plants, vegetables, berries, and sprouts. We were never designed to eat just meat (as mentioned, loaded with uric acid), especially the huge quantity of meat most Americans eat now at every single meal. Don't believe me? Why then do we not have fangs or any true canine teeth (like cats, dogs, bears, wolves, etc.) to tear and shred meat with? Why don't we have claws or other sharp appendages to fight and kill other animals? Why don't we have 4 legs to propel us fast enough to catch other fast animals? Why don't we have super keen sense of smell that most other predators have? And most importantly, why do humans have an incredibly long and twisted intestine and colon (obviously never meant to digest large quantities of meat)? Long before man evolved with his large brain and started developing spears, knives and other hunting tools, man lived primarily off of plants including vegetables, fruits, mushrooms, berries, and nuts. Coming back to present day, everyone knows that eating green leafy vegetables is healthy and the best source of nutrition, vitamins, calcium, minerals, and overall health, but it's astonishing how little greens are in most people's diets. Despite what most American school children think, ketchup is not a vegetable and neither are French fries or potato chips. The frozen vegetables people grab at the grocery or convenience stores and then microwave for dinner are not much better since they've been depleted of some of their vitamins, minerals and other nutritional content. A certain amount of raw, uncooked, unprocessed vegetables is key to long lasting health. This should include fresh salads, juiced vegetables (not store bought in a can), and some sort of green powdered drink, which will be discussed later in the book. I could list dozens of stories where acidic diets create havoc with people's bodies and their well-being, many of which were among the 16,500 people I spoke to at the Medco and Express Scripts table over the years. Here's one other shocking story, which I came across while working on a TV show. I met with a gorgeous girl named Stacey, who is strikingly beautiful and has a very lean body. Stacey mentioned that she was 5' 7" and weighed about 115 lbs. There was no indication that she had any health issues. It turns out that this 37 year 'young' girl has some allergies, but she also serious arthritis! In cold weather especially, it's troublesome as she does not have great circulation in her hands and feet and her doctor confirmed that she did in fact have arthritis. I asked if she'd ever seen photos of her blood (not just a typical blood report from the lab)? With new optical high definition microscopes, doctors can now see how healthy your blood is and get an idea if it is toxic and acidic, or healthy and slightly alkaline. I had a hunch that Stacey might have been eating a few acidic items on a regular basis. Turns out, she is a 'meat and potatoes' gal and eats red meat on a daily basis. She also eats potatoes, pasta, and drinks several sodas every day. While she does eat a limited amount of salads and vegetables, she admitted later that alkaline veggies do not make up even 50% of her diet. Having even a slightly acidic system is a recipe for disaster. Hopefully by the time you read this book, Stacey will have done the 7-Day "Alkalize & Energize" cleanse and finally decides to reclaim her health. I truly want to help people like Stacey and if we can help get rid of any signs of arthritis that she has now, we'll be sure to include that in the documentary film companion to this book. I had an extended interview with Dr. M. Phyllis Lose, the legendary equine veterinarian whose life is chronicled in the best selling book No Job For a Lady. Although Dr. Lose is in her 90's and technically retired, she is a model for perfect health as she already does most of the tips in this book. Up until two or three years ago she still worked vaccinating animals waking up Saturdays and Sundays at 4:30 am to work for her clients and making life pleasant for the thousands of animals (mostly horses) she has treated over her 60+ year career. When we started discussing diet and alkalinity, she brought up an interesting point that there was NO medical insurance for animals years ago, like there is today. Although there is now pet insurance (even for dogs and cats since they are now ironically getting affected by more cancer and terminal diseases), the owners of the horses Dr. Lose would examine including thoroughbreds for racing or breeding demanded the best food to ensure that their investment (these very expensive horses) stayed healthy. Dr. Lose performed many surgeries and in fact as the first female equine veterinarian in the U.S., she pioneered some of the modern day surgical techniques used today. Dr. Lose found the most effective way to keep a race horse healthy was to feed the horse a perfect blend of alfalfa, green timothy, and clover. The perfect blend of these highly alkaline grasses could slow down, and in many cases prevent arthritis and osteoporosis. Another interesting note is whenever the top racehorses got stomach ulcers (either from the stress of racing or the lactic acid that is physically produced inside the horse's body when racing), Dr. Lose had a fail proof solution. She would treat the horse with sodium bicarbonate (which is an alkaline drink - technically an antacid). Voila... after a few swigs of that sodium bicarbonate, the horse's ulcer would go away and often times any joint pain would subside very quickly. Referring specifically to the milk consumption in this country, higher milk consumption (with all that great calcium the American Dairy Association tell us to drink every day) actually leads to higher rates of osteoporosis as mentioned in a previous chapter. Part of this is due to the animal proteins and acids, which actually cause the body to leach calcium right out of the bones. The second problem is that even pure raw, organic milk from another animal species that has never been homogenized or pasteurized is not the best source of calcium. Just think about where the cow got the calcium in the first place? It was from the green grasses including the alkaline timothy, clover, and alfalfa. Humans can get great calcium right from the source from greens especially spinach, kale, wheat grass, etc. which are all alkaline. I can't begin to tell you how many people I've spoken to who walked up to the Express Scripts tables complaining of bone loss and osteoporosis. While most are older people in their 60's, 70's, and 80's, they have this blind faith that if they keep drinking 2 to 3 glasses of milk a day and take extra calcium pills, their bone density loss will stop or decrease. The only older people I've ever met with who seem exempt to any osteoporosis problems are vegetarians. If you've been losing bone density over the past few years and haven't been able to reverse or at least stop the loss, please research this acidity concept yourself. Doing the same thing over and over and expecting different results is the definition of insanity! The same goes for arthritis. It's been stated in many research articles that drinking milk can cause inflammation of the joints and lead to arthritis. Of course any other acidic foods or drinks like coffee, sodas, refined foods with sugars can also contribute to arthritis. Having any kind of joint pain, swelling, stiffness, and limited movement is a horrible way to live the final 20 to 30 years of your life. The good news is that more and more doctors and nutrition experts are proving that even rheumatoid arthritis (in which the body's own immune system starts to attack body tissues around joints) can be minimized and in many cases reversed with a proper alkaline diet and muscular therapy. Dr. Lose mentioned an interesting comment in passing that she has observed her entire career in treating thousands of animals. She stated (and this applies to people as well): "What keeps us alive is our strong immune system." Almost all doctors will agree that the quickest way to wreck havoc on your immune system by letting it become too acidic. After you finish reading this section you need to determine: Are you going to be among the 90% who take the Tums, the Alka-Seltzer, the Zantac or the Prilosec pill when you get the symptoms of acidity? Or are you going to be among the 10% who want to get to the root cause of these problems and properly alkalize, so that your immune system and all of your internal organs start working again in harmony at a balanced pH level? One medical professional (Patty Kay) I interviewed has seen just about every single illness and disease you could find in a hospital. She worked in a hospital as a registered nurse (R.N.) for almost 40 years. I met Patty and her daughter Vanessa on a commercial shoot where we spent the majority of the day discussing the importance of proper alkalinity. Patty and her daughter are both in amazing health as they are vegetarians and try to always eat organic. Patty recently quit the nursing industry out of frustration and disgust with the protocol that hospitals and doctors would issue to recovering cancer patients. Patty was flabbergasted that in this day and age, patients with cancer are given eggs, bacon, orange juice, coffee, toast, and jelly. While these items are part of the SAD ('Sad American Diet'), these are all acidic foods, which only add to the toxins already in the patient's bodies who were doing chemotherapy or radiation treatments. If

Patty were able to give advice to any of the patients, she would have recommended alkaline foods, vegetable juices, lemon water, and green tea. After seeing hundreds of patients die in the hospital while at the same time dozens of her friends outside the hospital doing holistic cancer treatments lived and thrived, she finally quit the nursing profession. There are hundreds of illnesses, diseases, and medical conditions that in most cases can be reversed or minimized with a properly balanced alkaline diet. If you contact the Gerson Institute directly, you'll see undisputed evidence of the worst cancer cases (sometimes stage III or stage IV) that have been treated successfully! I initially thought the title of Baroody's book Alkalize or Die was a little dramatic, but it isn't at all. If you prefer to watch documentary films, one of the best is by Ty Bollinger titled: "The Truth About Cancer." Keep reading and you'll understand that if you don't do the key things discussed in this book (most importantly getting rid of the excess acids and toxins in your system), you will have a much better chance of dying sooner rather than later!

ACTION ITEM 9.0

Identify and make a list of at least three acidic foods you realize you're eating every day. Decide today that you are going to eliminate or reduce at least one or two of these acidic foods and substitute some sort of alkaline food or drinks instead.

Chapter 10.
Sugar... The # 1 Addiction in the United States

Ask any nutritionist, homeopathic doctor, or chiropractor and they'll tell you sugar is the #1 cause of most health issues they see every day. Many medical doctors are now also beginning to see the plethora of negative effects from excess sugar intake including, but not limited to: perpetual food cravings, weight gain, obesity, Type II diabetes, cell inflammation, food allergies, mood swings, depression, lack of attention, trouble focusing, sleep deprivation, allergies, stress on the liver, and excess acid in the body which can directly cause ulcers, teeth decay, acid reflux, numerous diseases and cancer. BusinessInsider.com found that in 2010 the average American consumed over 100 lbs. of sugar every year! [10-1] WholeVegan.com did a more recent study which showed over 50% of Americans now eat 180 lbs. of sugar each year! That's quite an increase from the 18 lbs. of processed sugar people in this country consumed annually 200 years ago. It's easy to see how this is one of the biggest problems in the U.S. today. This sugar craze usually starts with getting children hooked on sugar – which most dietary experts agree is an 'addictive drug'. Children watching cartoons see dozens of cereal commercials every Saturday morning and when they travel in tow with their parents to the grocery store, many of the kid's cereals are located on the lower shelves easy for children to spot and grab. Some of those cereals have flashy mascots on the boxes or special toys inside to entice kids to beg their parents to get their favorite sugary, sweet cereals. Most parents would never dream of feeding Twinkies or several slices of chocolate fudge cake to their children first thing in the morning before school, but with some kid's cereals having 20 grams of sugar per serving, this is exactly what they're doing. I've witnessed children having at least two medium sized bowls of cereal - which would start your child off with 40 grams of sugar from the cereal alone. Flavored milk can add another 28 grams of sugar. If your child has juice, today's 'juice' drink' (often only 15% juice, but labeled similar to real juice and cheaper), that can add another 30 grams of sugar. Many of the children's vitamins now have glucose syrup or sorbitol (an added sugar substitute), so that's even more sugar! If your child just has just two bowls of cereal, some juice and a vitamin, he or she could easily start off the morning with almost 130 grams of sugar, let alone 500+ empty calories to help jump start child obesity. This is insanity! Sugar (and/or sugar substitutes) are now in almost every single food item you see in the grocery store. Just look at the following table to see how the sugar quickly adds up:

SERVING SIZE	BREAKFAST ITEM	AMOUNTof SUGAR:
1 bowl	Kellogg's Sugar Smacks cereal	20 grams
½ cup	flavored milk	28 grams
2nd bowl	Kellog's Sugar Smacks with milk	48 grams
1 carton	Juice 'Drink' beverage	30 grams
1 tablet	Multi-vitamin	3 grams
TOTAL	**ADDED SUGAR**	**129 grams**

This should be a wake up call for you and your children (if you have any), as the World Health Organization's daily recommended daily intake of sugar for adults is 25 grams! Of course this assumes your child doesn't add a couple of slices of toast (with artificial butter and sugar laden jelly) or have a few pancakes or waffles soaked with sugary syrup. This also assumes your kid is not one of the millions of kids who grabs a soda and candy bar from the school vending machines later that morning when the first sugar crash hits a few hours after his or her 'nutritional' breakfast. No wonder the Centers for Disease Control in back in 2011 classified 17% of American children as obese, and some new studies have estimated 33% of teenagers and adolescents are now obese. A big part of this is due to excess caloric intake and excess sugar. Many experts are seriously concerned that this obesity number could approach 50% of all American children in the next five to ten years! A recent Pediatrics report found that overall, half of overweight teens and have one or more risk factors for heart disease, diabetes, high blood pressure, or high levels of bad cholesterol. [10-2] They say a picture is worth a thousand words, so here's a visual analogy how sugar burns in the human body... think about an open campfire with a flame going. If you poured gasoline directly on that fire, those flames would immediately flare up providing you with beautiful colors with lots of light and warmth for a few seconds, and then the flames would quickly die down. That gasoline is similar to you slugging a sugar-laden soda. You'll immediately get a great sugar high and feel great for a few minutes from that sweet soda, but it won't last long. Now visualize the fire again... if you've placed some small kindling (my favorite is tiny dead pine branches with lots of bark and sap) on your fire, this too will flame up almost like gasoline giving you a large bright flame, lots of heat for a few minutes longer this time, but eventually the fire will die down. The only way to build a long lasting, steady fire is once the fire is going, you need to add some large logs (dry, 'dead' oak is particularly good) that will burn slow and steady to last a long time. The next time you're sitting by a campfire or even near a regular fireplace, notice the size of the logs that burn the longest. They are usually the largest and most solid logs. Now let's look at the calories (FYI...calories like the fire represent heat energy that your body burns) you're putting into your body every day. If you're eating foods with high sugar content, you're definitely experiencing sugar highs and lows, let alone all the long-term health risks. Why not visualize the steady, long burning fireplace and give your body the long lasting fuel (protein and carbohydrates, with a small mix of natural fats and sugar) to perform consistently. A few examples of breakfast foods that have much lower sugar content (or at least natural sugar which is healthier) would include: organic almond milk, 100% vegetable or fruit juice, organic eggs, nuts, sprouts, wheat toast (without jelly), vegetables, or fruit (a limited amount as most fruit is high in sugar). Think of these types of natural foods as healthy 'logs' that will fuel your body for many hours. This is the proper way to fuel your body for slow, steady, reliable energy all day long. The biggest question I get from friends, clients, etc. once they discover how bad sugar is for their health is: "How can I get off the addiction of sugar?". I remind them that their massive daily sugar intake didn't happen overnight, and tell them that it's a gradual process. Take small steps every day to cut back on the highest sugar content foods such as donuts, pastries, desserts, candy bars, etc. Also, it's best not to quit sugar cold turkey, as your body might have adverse reactions. If you're currently used to an afternoon snack of a Coke and chocolate chip cookie, 'substitute' a green tea and a banana. Slowly transition your snacks towards healthier versions with natural sugar and eventually little or no sugar. One of the other habits I suggest is to always have a large glass of alkaline, lemon water in front of you, or some kind of green drink. If you're always sipping water, it helps fill you up so that you don't seem quite as hungry and the psychological impact of constantly sipping water will take your focus away from wanting as much sugar. While working on this chapter this morning, I've already slugged down 3 large lemon waters and 2 green drinks. I feel no hunger and have tons of energy. The more healthy foods and drinks you keep substituting, the healthier and more energetic you will feel...I promise! Also make sure you do the below action assignment tonight or as soon as you're able to. I think you'll find the film enjoyable and extremely enlightening if you haven't seen it yet.

ACTION ITEM 10.0
Rent, stream or download the movie "Fed Up." Film critics agree this is the most powerful film ever done revealing the *true* facts about sugar!

Chapter 11.
The KEY? Proper Alkalinity Balance

While I've been doing many years of research for several health books now and working on the companion feature length documentary film "The Health Pill" (which hopefully will be released in a year or two), the best introduction I got to the importance of alkalinity was from my friend Tony Robbins. Tony has an audio program called "Get the Edge" and one of the sessions is all about proper alkalinity and how it changed his life and his understanding of energy, health, disease and cancer. I strongly recommend his program "Get the Edge" at his website, Amazon or you may be able to find it at your local library. It's the most logical, simple, and profound introduction to this critically important topic. Tony is a master at synthesizing information (in this case from doctors, nutritionists, and other health experts) and explaining the subject in layman's terms. In addition I learned a great deal about the importance of proper alkalinity from researching Dr. Max Gerson and his daughter Charlotte Gerson (who continued in his foot steps with The Gerson Clinic), and Dr. Robert Young who has made pH balance one of his cornerstones of health when talking to his patients. As mentioned earlier, I admit to being so focused with this concept of proper alkalinity that I got an A+ tattooed on my arm. I think my fascination began when I first saw Hollywood stars (even some of the middle aged actors in their 50's and 60's) who had incredible physiques. You can probably picture a lean body with well proportioned muscles and a flat abdomen with the famous 'six-pack'. As I started getting involved with Hollywood and working with some of these stars, not only were they truly in great shape (remember the camera adds 15 lbs.), but most of these folks had incredible energy. Whenever I had the opportunity, I'd ask what they were doing and most would say they train or work out on a regular basis, but I found out years later that most of them also had a nutritionist, a dietician and a strict daily diet or lifestyle that they adhered to most of the time. It wasn't until years later in my 40's that I found out this secret of alkalinity. I'm in my 50's now and it doesn't do me any good to have six-pack abs (even though ironically I finally got them!) for middle- aged roles and nobody would want to see my pasty-white stomach in the first place since I don't tan very well. But here's the point... I really don't care about the six-pack and the super lean body I easily achieved when I found out this secret of an alkaline lifestyle, but perhaps if you're an actor, a model, or a young person who just wants to look great in a bathing suit, this information will help you. For me, the reason I became so excited about this concept of proper alkalinity is I no longer have to carry around the extra five to ten lbs. of weight I had for about 20 years. Even though I was never considered fat or felt overweight at all, the elimination of those last ten lbs. has made me run faster, hike up hills almost effortlessly, walk easier, and simply have more energy! Even if you don't need to lose any weight, who doesn't want to have more energy and feel better? The other main benefit is I never get sick anymore and haven't caught as much as a head cold in the last fifteen years. If I feel the slightest bit out of whack, or feel a cold or fever coming on, I'll drink an abundance of alkaline water or green drink and within 24 hours my body is back in balance and I'm feeling great again. Paul Gunn is a high-energy stunt man, model and actor who looks and 'acts' ten years younger than his real age. I worked a live event with Paul last year in Las Vegas and after each ten-hour day, Paul raced off to his other 'night job', which was jumping over galloping horses, chasing down other soldiers and getting into spectacular sword fights. His other gig was at the 'Tournament of Kings' live dinner show at the Excalibur Hotel & Casino. Paul knows about the importance of a proper alkaline diet and lifestyle and when he works he complements this by drinking alkaline water. Paul is now a spokesperson for Real Water - which is super alkaline, antioxidant water celebrities and athletes enjoy. I know it's real and part of his regimen because I've witnessed Paul in high-energy mode for 18 hours at both his day and night jobs (for this one week anyway) and he always has a bottle with him. If interested you can find Real Water at most Costco stores or at www.drinkrealwater.com. My company, Nemours Marketing did our own follow up research (from dozens of books, research papers, hundreds of our own interviews) before sharing our own 7-Day "Alkalize & Energize" cleanse now with over 500 success stories to date. Some of those amazing results are shared in this book. As mentioned, 7.36 is the ideal pH level your body should be (which is slightly alkaline), or your body will literally start breaking itself down, leading to illness, disease, and possibly cancer. Healthy, alkaline cells have lots of electrons (which provide electrical energy) and ensure a negative charge on the outside of your red blood cells, which help them move swiftly and efficiently through your blood stream. As mentioned, Dr. Robert Young wrote a comprehensive book on this subject called The pH Miracle. What Dr. Young shares from his research is that obese people are often times over-acid. On CNN, he showed remarkable photos of some of his patients who've lost over 100 lbs. and are now the epitome of perfect health. More and more doctors like Dr. Leonard Coldwell (www.DrLeonardColdwell.com) are stating that cancer can be stopped completely by properly alkalizing your body. Tony Robbins himself is the poster boy for perfect health as he spends as many as 275 days on the road each year meeting tens of thousands of people at his live events. You couldn't be more exposed to more germs or potentially sick people than Tony, yet he consistently has such incredible energy and has never been sick in over 25 years! Tony attributes his incredible energy, vitality, and health to his alkaline diet and lifestyle. I've been fortunate in the same way. Over the past two decades when attending the different Health Benefit Fairs for Medco and Express Scripts, I'm usually on the road non-stop for two to three months. I sometimes travel between two or three cities in a single day and the weather can vary 30 to 50 degrees depending on which cities I'm passing through. On top of the crowded airports, I often interact with hundreds of people (including a few who are sick). Yet, knock on wood, I've never gotten sick in over 15 years! My simple analogy of the importance of 7.36 pH alkalinity is the 98.6° F temperature that your body should function at. If you're outside on a very hot day, certain body functions will slow down, blood flow to your extremities will increase, and your body will start sweating. On a cold day, your body will limit the amount of blood flowing to your outer epidermis (your skin) and eventually your muscles will contract as you start shivering. This involuntary action of shivering is to keep your body moving and therefore warm your body. This is also a warning signal to do something like light a fire, find shelter, or add clothing to warm your body up. Your body is smart enough to also warn you of increased acidity. If your body falls much below the magic 7.36 pH balance level, you can get ulcers, acid reflux, stomach aches, feel fatigued, just to name a few warning signals. It's ridiculous to keep ignoring these signals to the body! The long-term solution is not just to take more Tums, Alka-Seltzer, or Prilosec. This would be like driving your car and when the 'check engine' light comes on, instead of changing the motor oil and filters, you instead cut the little wire to the dashboard light and keep on driving. Sooner or later you're going to have to pay the piper. This is exactly what happens if you ignore the signals of an acidic body. In just a few months, or a few years disease could appear or worse, some kind of cancer could manifest when often it's too late. Just like battery acid that sometimes spills onto your battery post and starts corroding your car's battery terminals, too much acid in your body will start corroding your organs and disrupting all kinds of body functions leading to a complete breakdown of normal body functions as you'll learn in the next chapter. In 1994, Dr. Young discovered the biological transformation of red blood cells into bacteria in acidic environments. Dr. Young and his wife Shelley are alkalinity experts and have written many other books on the subject of alkalinity and Ph balance. Their noble life mission is to do all they can to change lives and save lives with an alkaline lifestyle and diet. Finally almost 3 decades later for his ground breaking work on alkalinity, Dr. Young is starting to get the respect he deserves from some of his peers such as this quote from Neil Solomon, M.D., PhD: "Dr. Young may be on the threshold of a new biology whose principles will revolutionize the biology and medicine worlds."

One final inspirational story to share that will hopefully have an impact on anyone who has ever had acne problems or skin issues. This includes the millions of teenagers who battle acne on a daily basis. I was working on the TV show "Scorpion" a few years ago and met a very talented actress and stand up comedian named Vanessa Esperanza. We got to chatting about health and even though Vanessa was very beautiful, she wanted to try out the 7-Day "Alkalize & Energize" Cleanse to lose a few lbs., boost her energy and see if she could clear up her skin.

Fast forward a few days later and here's the e-mail she sent:

"Scott, I want to thank you for introducing this to me! My skin is much better just after 1 week! I noticed little breakouts on my chin but the big hormonal acne on my cheeks has gone way down! I also was fighting a cold when I started this and that was wild. I had cold like symptoms but felt healthy! No aches, lots of energy, my throat was scratchy but no pain at all! And I was better by day 3."

An exciting update on Vanessa as this book goes to press. She met her Prince Charming and I just got word last week that she is engaged. Congratulations Vanessa!

I've also worked with several young people and teenagers who have cleared up their acne within 7 to 14 days and I would never promise anyone or guarantee that this cleanse would eliminate the serious hormonal acne many teenagers struggle with, but think about it this way. If your face is erupting, this may be a sign that you have internal toxins which your body is desperately trying to expel through your epidermis. If you look at the horrible diet of most teenagers including pizza, potato chips, fast foods, processed foods, sodas and energy drinks, cleansing out your system along with drinking an abundance of water would very likely help. Please pass this info along to any teenagers you may know!

ACTION ITEM 11.0
Find a pH chart at your local health food store or on-line today which will show you a comprehensive list of alkaline and acidic foods. Then make a decision to start balancing your pH through more alkaline foods and beverages.

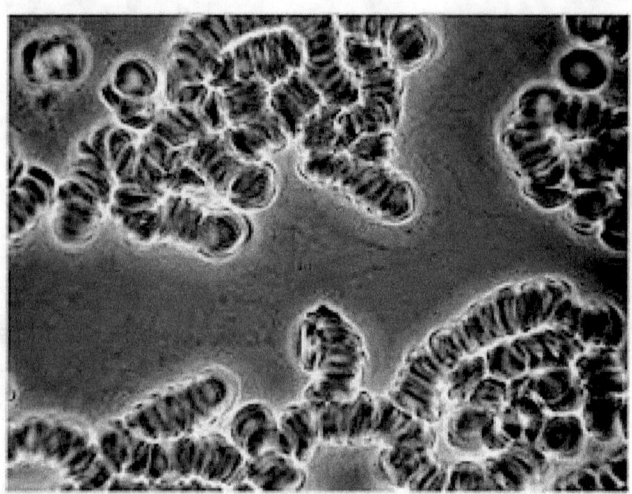

'Acidic' blood showing red blood cells clumped together
reducing the effective transport of oxygen. The dark
spots are candida (yeast), bacteria, and fungus
developing in this toxic environment.
(photo courtesy of NaturalFatLoss.com)

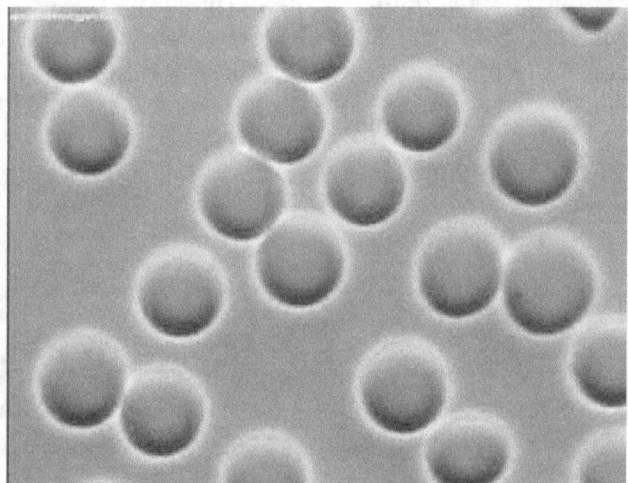

An 'alkaline' environment. The red blood cells are perfectly
round & plump. The alkaline, electric charge outside cells helps
them move rapidly to carry lots of oxygen without sticking to
each other. Notice also how clean the blood is!
(photo courtesy of NaturalFatLoss.com)

Chapter 12.
Energize!

Do you ever look at certain people and wonder: "Wow...where did they get all their energy?" I used to wonder when I' d see someone like Jack LaLanne or Tony Robbins. I'd say to myself: "I wish I had all the amazing energy he has!" I've heard all kinds of explanations including: "He was probably born an energetic person", or "His father had the same intense energy... it must be in the genes." I used to believe the nonsense that massive energy was reserved for the 'chosen few' or that certain people were born with more energy. The truth is YOU create your own energy! Barring certain diseases or medical issues, there are very specific, detailed steps almost anyone can take to dramatically increase their energy level and I'm not talking about a temporary caffeine or energy-drink boost either. I'm talking about serious long-term, steady energy that will keep you going all day long while having the ability to live life to the fullest including achieving your goals and dreams. So what's the secret? What are the specific steps one needs to take to realize a dramatic boost in their energy? The first and most important step is the fuel (food) you put into your body every day. Nobody with a high performance sports car would ever think about putting cheap (low octane) gasoline in their car. Most people gladly spend a little extra to get the higher octane, higher quality fuel so their car engine performs better, more smoothly and gets improved fuel economy. In the case of your body, the secret is to eat energy-laden foods! I already mentioned the importance of alkalinity, but it's equally important that most of your food intake has real energy. Remember that every organ in your body (starting with your heart) needs electrical energy to function and keep you alive and healthy. Bear with me for a moment, as I break down this concept in very simple terms. If you examine the cells inside your body (all health starts at the cellular level), you will find that human cells operate optimally at a high vibration energy frequency of 60 to 80 megahertz (MHz).[12-1] It's common sense that we should consume foods that have a natural vibration energy (electrical life force) closest to that of our own cells. The highest-vibration, life force energy foods are raw fruits and vegetables, especially those full of the sun's natural energy such as chlorophyll-rich leafy greens. There are several ways to measure this electrical energy from foods now including special Kirlian photography and the BT3 frequency monitoring system created by Mr. Bruce Tainio of Tainio Technology. There are dozens of studies and papers that discuss the electrical energy from different foods, but the best list I've seen in terms of including different alkaline vegetables and fruits we should be eating to begin with, I complied from Tony Robbins' "Get the Edge" program. By the way, if you're serious about mastering this concept of having a LOT more energy, I strongly recommend you attend Tony's live 'Unleash the Power Within' live seminar, which includes a full day health event called 'The Power of Pure Energy'. I promise this seminar will change every aspect of your life! OK, enough of the commercial, below is a table I assembled using information from Robbins Research Institute, GreenandJuicy.com, and Tanio Technology [12-2] :

SAMPLE FOODS AND THEIR 'ENERGY' MEASUREMENTS

FOOD	ELECTRICAL ENERGY
chocolate cake	1 - 3 MHz
hamburger	5 MHz
raw almonds	40 – 50 MHz
raw green vegetables	70 – 90 MHz
wheat grass	70 – 90 MHz
lavender oil	118 MHz
lentil sprouts	150 MHz
live roses	320 MHz

Note that the electrical vibrational energy of the human body (and most human organs) is 62 to 72 MHz. Common sense should dictate that if most of your diet is junk food (5 MHz or less), or processed or packaged foods (also low energy), or if all of your food is microwaved or cooked (drastically reduced electrical energy), you will suffer from low energy. By eating real, whole foods and making sure that at least some of your food intake is raw (ex: salads, raw veggies, sprouts, juices, nuts), your body will run at peak efficiency and you will have a lot more energy! Once again, I'm talking about sustained, long-term energy where you feel good for hours on end. Not a quick sugar or caffeine buzz like you might get from a can of cola. To measure exactly how much energy someone gains from changing their diet is very subjective as there are other factors and it's often hard to quantify how much extra energy someone has from changing their diet to include more live, alkaline, electrical foods (mostly green vegetables). However, I'd like to share four specific examples of people I've worked with or encountered who have experienced massive increases in their energy levels:

1) **Ronald Farnham** (in his late 30's) massively boosted his energy after he first completed our 7-Day "Alkalize & Energize" cleanse and later changed his daily diet to almost all raw, alkaline vegetables. Ronald had this to share: "The most important benefit to me was my energy level at the end of the 90 days, which went through the roof. I've always been a night person when writing my screenplays and books, and in the six months after cleansing my system, I was writing like a machine until 3 or 4 in the morning. In those six months, I finished writing three books (all now are published) and completed four screenplays, one of which ("Hollywood + Vine") will go into production next month. I also had the energy to write, direct, produce, and edit 20 episodes of my own web series called "The Ronald Show". While I'm proud of these accomplishments this past year, the specific reason I mention this is these creative tasks take a great deal of time and energy and I doubt I would be getting this much work done if I hadn't cleansed my system."

2) **Nick Yaya** (in his early 40's) started with the "Alkalize & Energize" cleanse and from there transitioned into a healthy, daily lifestyle which includes juicing or vegetable-fruit smoothies every morning. His new healthy lifestyle he's maintained consists of a lot more alkaline, energetic foods including more vegetables. There was a six-month period between the time I last saw the 'old' Nick and when I saw the 'new' Nick, and I had to do a double take, as he had lost 35 lbs! In addition to his new, slim physique, Nick's skin now looks very smooth and vibrant (almost glowing), and his facial features including his jaw line are more pronounced and distinct. Since Nick is a Hollywood

actor, this is a big benefit to him and you can see the results below in his 'before' and 'after' commercial headshots showing a more youthful and energetic look.

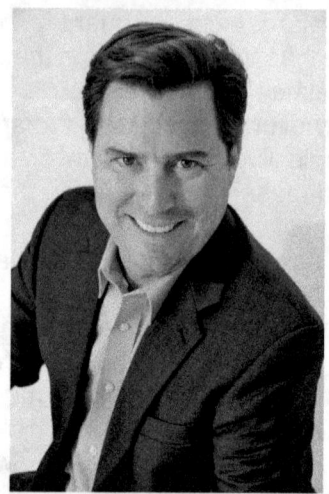

Nick 'before'

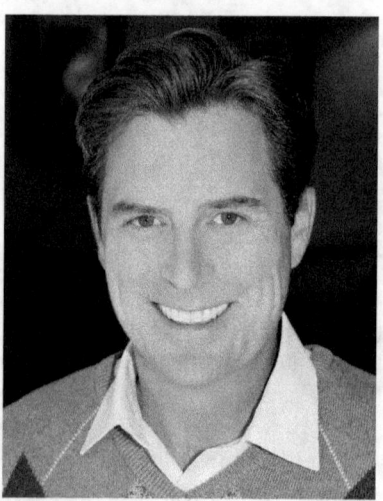

Nick's 'after' shot where he is
actually several years older.

Without having to carry around the extra 35 lbs. and with his increased energy levels, Nick is now able to juggle more work, tackle more auditions, master his acting classes, and has even found extra time and energy to follow his dreams. Nick is going out on more auditions than ever, getting invited to more call-backs from different casting directors, and booking more work (like the lead role on an independent film he landed this week). A side benefit is that Nick also got off of his prescriptions that his doctor had previously told him he'd "have to take the rest of his life". Congratulations Nick!

3) **Jim Britton** is a 75-year-old gentleman I met at a health benefits fair in New Mexico. Jim appears to be about 65 years old and is very fit and trim. By changing his diet over the last six months, he dropped 30 lbs. (went from 190 down to 160) and lost 4" in his waistline. Jim decided to cut out all breads & wheat products, and is now eating a lot more vegetables along with his new favorite fruit... avocados. With these new energetic foods that Jim is eating on a regular basis, he feels much better and mentioned that he "now enjoys an abundance of natural energy!" You really notice his energy as well as he is now the type of individual you look at and remark: "Wow... I wish I had all of his energy."

4) **Desmond Bailey** is a friend I've known for many years. We met on set of the TV show "Rizzoli and Isles" as we were both booked as regular Detectives on the show. One day Desmond overheard me talking about the 7 -Day "Alkalize & Energize" cleanse and he was very skeptical to say the least. Then one day (about five years ago) he decided to give the cleanse a go and what happened during those first seven days changed his life. Desmond's blood pressure started at 151/87 and ended at 125/75. His total cholesterol started up at 232 and dropped to 198. In those seven days he lost 12 lbs. and for the first time in almost 20 years, he "has never felt better and had as much energy". He was also thrilled to eventually (a few months later) get off all of his prescription drugs. When I see Desmond from time to time, he looks about five to ten years younger and weighs in at 180 lbs. vs. the 215 lbs. he used to weigh several years ago. He always thanks me for helping him transition into a healthy lifestyle after the cleanse, which he says was the catalyst for his new life! On the opposite side of the energy spectrum, I once had a roommate (I won't mention his name), who was the most

lethargic person I'd ever met. Even though he slept a full eight to ten hours each night, he always seemed tired. His diet was almost all processed or packaged, and often frozen foods (including microwaveable dinners), meats and cheeses. He drank lots of Gatorade, lemonade, soda, and juice-drinks (less than 10% real juice). With all of that acidic, sugar ladened, 'dead' food and almost no live, green vegetables, it's not hard to understand where his lack of energy stemmed from. So, how is your energy level? If you don't have the high energy levels you desire, take an honest look at the food you're eating on a regular basis. Are you eating mostly live, energetic foods? If not, take the challenge below. Although there are many other tips for boosting your energy (such as moving your body, improving your posture, super-hydrating with alkaline water, and improving your psychology, which I'll cover later in this book), fueling yourself with energetic food is the most important tip and the most logical place to start! Don't forget to consume energetic beverages as well including plenty of alkaline water and green drinks!

ACTION ITEM 12.0
Write a list of all the foods and drinks that pass through your lips the next 24 hours. Assess what kind of electrical energy those food have and decide today to either start with a cleanse, or take the important step to start eating or drinking at least 1 or 2 energetic foods today to boost your energy!

Chapter 13.
The Vegetarian Trend

As an actor, I'm always observing people very carefully. I look at people's outer appearance and skin (since that's what the camera sees) and over the past few years I have this uncanny ability to accurately guess who is a vegetarian most of the time. One day I was working on a TV game show "The Pyramid" that my friend Mike Richards was producing and hosting. I was sitting in the audience next to a beautiful girl named Dianne who was very pretty and had absolutely flawless, silky smooth skin. I figured she was in her mid 30's. Dianne was telling me stories about her world travels, her different careers, and then she started going on and on about her tours in Vietnam as a nurse. This girl (actually a middle aged lady) had done two tours in Vietnam! She was actually 25+ years older than she looked! The only thing Dianne told me that did not shock me was that she had become a vegetarian 30 years ago.

While I'm not 100% vegetarian (or a vegan), I applaud the growing number of vegetarians for several reasons. Eating fresh vegetables, fruits, sprouts, nuts, etc. is a very healthy lifestyle as it is food in its most natural state. Almost every vegetarian I've met (including Dianne) looks healthy, appears energetic, and usually has glowing, radiant skin. In addition to hydrating by drinking lots of water, vegetarians are getting a large quantity of water (in essence hydrating) through all the water-rich vegetables, fruits, and sprouts they eat. I've shifted my diet the past few years to 90% vegetarian and in addition to alkalizing my body with natural, alkaline vegetarian foods, I'm by default hydrating my cells every time I eat water-rich veggies and fruits. If you don't have any close family members or friends who are vegetarians, or if you think that vegetarians are unhealthy or simply crazy, don't be too quick to judge. Some of the most energetic and healthy people I've ever met or worked with are vegetarians or vegans. There are hundreds of famous people you probably know or have seen on screen including: Ryan Seacrest, Kate Winslet, Paul McCartney, Leonardo

DiCaprio, Alexandra Paul, Elizabeth Berkley, Christian Bale, Tobey Maguire, James Cameron, Tony Robbins, Bill Clinton, Natalie Portman, and Brad Pitt. You'd also be surprised at the list of hundreds of professional athletes as well including: Heisman trophy winner Ricky Williams, Atlanta Falcons tight end Tony Gonzalez, legendary tennis champion Chris Everett, UFC champion Mac Danzig, and NY Jets icon Joe Namath. Dr. William Casteli of the Framingham Heart Study reported in his study: "Vegetarians have the lowest cholesterol counts, and the lowest rates of cancer and heart disease. Those with the lowest cholesterol levels also outlived everyone else." [13-1] The main concern uneducated people have about going vegetarian, is that they think they can't get enough nutrition or protein. I strongly suggest you research how much protein you can get from different all-natural sources including spinach, kale, mushrooms, sprouts, and of course nuts. There's no way in this short book I can get into all the details, but there are books out there as well as information on-line where you can get more info, including great menus if this is a lifestyle you end up choosing. As mentioned, I've never felt better since 90% of my diet is alkaline consisting of primarily water-rich vegetarian foods. I occasionally eat meat when offered to me on special social occasions including the Holidays, but I almost never buy or prepare any meat dishes myself. The other reason to consider being a vegetarian (besides being great for your health) is for the health of our planet. With the rapidly growing population and limited resources, climate change, etc. we're all going to face more food and water shortages if we continue the course we're on. There are several great documentaries out including: "Last Call at the Oasis" and "Tapped" which explore how severe this water problem is becoming. I'd also suggest reading one of John Robbins' best selling books, either: May All Be Fed or The Food Revolution. In these books, the passionate author (who was constantly sick as a child eating lots of his family's Baskin-Robbins ice cream as well as meat, cheese, etc.), not only talks about how he found true health, but John shares compelling information about how inefficient (and what a waste of resources) it is for us to eat a meat-favored diet vs. a plant-based diet. Consider this mind-blowing statistic straight from the Water Education Foundation. It takes 2,464 gallons of water to produce 1 lb.

of California beef, while it only takes 23 gallons of water to produce 1 lb. of lettuce! [13-2]. This is an insane and unsustainable way to feed the world especially with millions of new meat lovers around the world (including the booming populations of China and other Asian countries) switching from a vegetable and rice-based diet to fast food and meat-based diets. As you may have read, there are thousands of new McDonald's and Burger King restaurants being added every year overseas. By the way, the health of the Chinese population (while not nearly as bad as it is here in America) is declining fast including millions of new cases of Type II diabetes being reported in China alone each year! The final reason to consider going vegetarian (or vegan) is that vegetarians live an average of six to ten years longer than the rest of the population! [13-3] If you're still not sold on eating more veggies, please read and ponder this quote from one of the smartest men in the history of the world. Albert Einstein had the foresight many years to ago to write: "Nothing will benefit human health and increase the chances for survival of life on earth as much as the evolution of a vegetarian diet". Now that was one smart man!

ACTION ITEM 13.0

Do your own research about vegetarians. If you're not a vegetarian already and end up liking the results of your research, consider at least shifting more towards a plant-based diet and cutting out some meat from your current lifestyle.

Chapter 14.
Diets: Fad or Fiction?

According to Merriam-Webster, one of the definitions of diet is: "a regimen of eating and drinking sparingly so as to reduce one's weight (ex. going on a diet)". It seems every few months, somebody is coming out with some new fad diet or diet book. I don't think ANY diet is a long term, sustainable healthy way of life. Look at the first three letters of diet... D.I.E.! That ought to tell you something. In the last 40 years there have been numerous diets and/or diet supplements that have generated lots of publicity to sell more books or supplement products, but were later proven to be unhealthy. In 1977, Slim Fast was introduced. In 1979 Dexatrim became a hit before the ingredient PPA was linked to a risk of stroke. In the 1990's, there was the 'low fat' diet which had it's own problems, in 1992 there was the 'Atkins' diet which promoted super-high protein and low carbohydrates. In 2004, Ephedra was a popular supplement until there was a correlation to possible heart attacks. One of the newer and trendy diets now is the 'Paleo' (or Caveman) diet, which is a fairly common sense approach (except in my opinion it's a little heavy on the meats). Of course, there are 'low sugar' diets, which promote Aspartame (one of the most common artificial sweeteners in use today) which has it's own potential negative side effects. There are hundreds of reports and articles showing the dismal failure of people in the U.S. who try diets, but the failure rate is just as bad overseas. Some 34 million Britons embarked on diets last year - but an astonishing 99% eventually piled the weight they lost back on.[14-1] While a temporary fast for a day or two, or a multi-day cleanse is fine, any diet which restricts or minimizes your daily caloric intake is not a good long term approach. It's likely that you'll deprive your body of the nutrients that you need. It's common sense that we should adopt a long term, healthy lifestyle with the proper daily caloric intake and at least 80% of all foods being healthy and all natural. Your body was designed to operate and function in a healthy manner from natural, organic foods that come from the earth, not from a pill, can, box, or shrink-wrapped. We were certainly not designed to follow a strictly regulated diet with rules that don't usually make common sense.

ACTION ITEM 14.0

Do your own research on the high failure rates of diets and decide today instead of trying any 'diet', you're going to transition to better 'habits' & a long term lifestyle of eating a sensible amount of more healthy, all-natural foods.

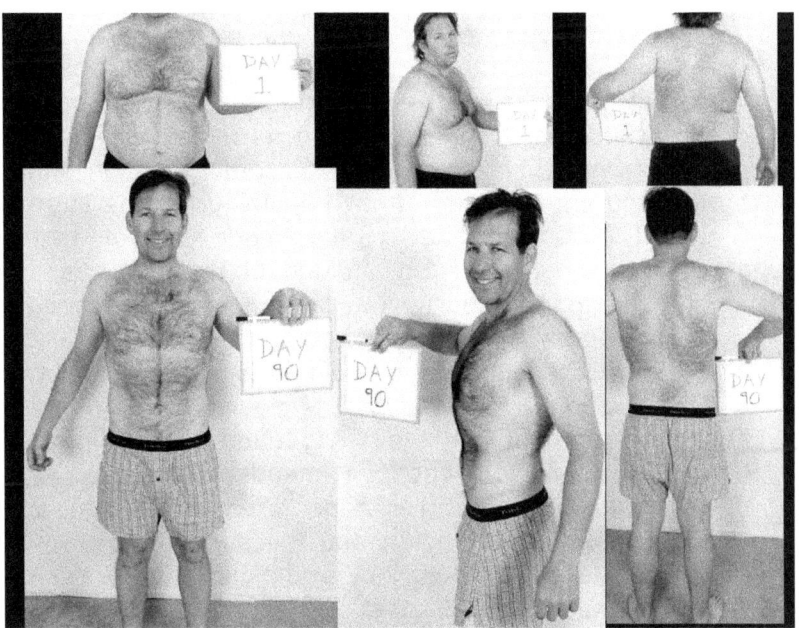

No Fiction here! This was Ronald on Day 1 and Day 90
after he transitioned to a healthy lifestyle!

Chapter 15.
Secrets for a Healthy Mouth and Teeth

You've probably heard the old saying: "Watch out, that sugar will rot your teeth!" This is a misnomer, as sugar does not actually rot teeth. Ask any dentist or dental hygienist and they'll tell you it's the sugar "when it metabolizes into acid" that actually rots your teeth. This acid problem (discussed at great length in a previous chapter), reinforces the fact that you must watch your pH levels and work on consuming more alkaline foods and drinks for your overall health. A slightly alkaline diet is just as important if you want to enjoy your own teeth for your entire life. It's common for archeologists to excavate human remains thousands of years old and when looking at the skulls, they often find ancient teeth in perfect condition with no holes or cavities! A primary reason is that early homo sapiens did not have anything like the current Standard American Diet (SAD) made up of highly processed and refined foods along or twenty times the amount of sugar! In addition to all the modern acidic foods, if you add in all the sugary, sweetened beverages along with the modern staples of coffee, energy drinks, and sodas (all acidic), you'll realize it is playing havoc with the health of your mouth and the strength and longevity of your teeth. The final straw (no pun intended) is people who drink alcohol on a regular basis. Remember that any alcoholic drink is very acidic and that's why many winos and drunks lose their teeth. Any acidic drinks will over time wear the enamel off your teeth as well. Your dentist has probably given you some great additional advice, but it seems like many people don't take heed, so here's a reminder: brush your teeth (with a soft bristled brush) at least twice a day, floss often, and use some sort of mouthwash to fight gingivitis and gum disease. I admit there are people blessed with slightly stronger teeth and bones than others, but here are seven specific tips that will improve the overall health of your mouth and help you retain your full set of adult teeth:

1) Drink lots of water (alkaline water or drinks are best).

2) Rinse your mouth with water after eating or drinking anything.

3) Get a WaterPik or similar type of water flossing system (it's much easier and quicker than traditional flossing) and use twice a day on low or medium pressure, or occasionally in between flossing.

4) Invest in a metal tongue sweeper (about $12) to skim oral bacteria and food debris off your tongue. This will help eliminate bad breath and minimize the acidic breeding ground in the middle of your mouth.

5) Make your own toothpaste by mixing 3 parts baking soda and 1 part hydrogen peroxide. Brush your teeth and gums gently to clean your mouth and help whiten your teeth.

6) Make your own mouthwash by mixing 1 part water and 3 parts hydrogen peroxide. Gargle throughout your whole mouth and feel the peroxide working it's magic! Afterwards, rinse your mouth with water.

7) Always be careful about biting too hard on solid food objects that could damage or wear down your teeth.

Of course, the most important reminder is the less acidic (more alkaline) your diet, the better health for your mouth and you'll have a much better chance of keeping all your teeth in excellent condition! I've been following these tips for years and although I might just be lucky, I'm also grateful to have never had a cavity! If my track record doesn't 100% convince you that you can ensure perfect teeth by adjusting your diet, there was a remarkable find recently with new high-tech scans of Pompeii residents killed in the eruption of Mount Vesuvius. "The ancient Romans had perfect teeth thanks to healthy, low-sugar diet. The population had amazing teeth thanks to a low-sugar, high-fiber Mediterranean diet. The inhabitants of Pompeii ate a lot of fruit and vegetables but very little sugar", a dental expert tells the Telgraph.[15-1] It's interesting that over 2,000 years ago, even without fancy toothpastes, mouthwashes, expensive dental procedures, etc. that common sense and healthy food allowed many people to maintain and enjoy perfect, complete healthy sets of teeth their entire lives.

ACTION ITEM 15.0

In addition to focusing on more alkaline foods and drinks, start a habit today to rinse your mouth with water after every meal or snack. In addition to better overall mouth health, by getting rid of loose food particles, you'll notice better breath and less chance of acidification in your mouth that could damage your teeth and your smile.

Chapter 16.
Warning... Obesity Now Declared a Disease!

With over 1/3rd of Americans labeled obese and many more overweight, it's become common-place (the new normal) to be a little overweight. The American Medical Association has now labeled Obesity as an official disease! It's no big deal to be just a few pounds overweight right? Wrong... being overweight and/or obese is linked to increased risk of heart disease, Type II diabetes, high blood pressure, certain cancers, and many other chronic conditions. In fact, in the U.S. alone, overweight and obesity are correlated with many of these leading causes of death and may decrease your lifespan by 5 to 20 years! [16-1] Instead of making this a lengthy chapter on the many different medical complications and terrible side effects being overweight can lead to, I'd rather inspire you with a few people who have shed weight fairly quickly and totally turned their lives around. The first is Ronald Farnham (mentioned earlier) who wrote the introduction for my first health book. Ronald's story is pretty incredible shedding 60 pounds in 90 days and in the process gaining so much energy, he appeared to be almost super human. Ronald became a successful (and very prolific) writer and now is even a film producer. Tosca Reno has been called the 'Comeback Covergirl'. Tosca is now 57 years 'young' and just a few years ago when most ladies hang up their sneakers and stop going to the gym, she became dissatisfied with the 70 extra lbs. she was lugging around every day. She went from exhausted and overweight to vibrant and ripped, and even became a fitness model! Beyond the physical changes, Ms. Reno also transformed her relationship with food, becoming a certified nutritionist and embracing an 'Eat-Clean' philosophy. Now she' s devoted to helping others find their way through her blog, consulting, and writing 15 health books including The Start Here Diet. Instead of sitting quietly on the couch, Reno is speaking up as a regular guest on shows like "Dr. Oz", "Good Morning America", and "The Doctors".[16-2] If you're close to retirement age and want to be inspired, read the AARP article footnoted below about Tosca. Charles Ellington was an indirect client of mine. He was coached by my good friend Bruce Ellington (Charles' son) who also had tremendous success when I first met him doing our 7-Day "Alkalize & Energize" cleanse. Mr. Ellington, a retired Tuskegee airman was 89 at the time and with the coaching and support of his Bruce and his wife lost 55 lbs. in less than 6 months. While it's always better to prevent the added weight early on, or catch kids and teens early, Charles proved it's never too late to drop the weight and re-gain excellent health! I've worked with many individuals who have lost 10 lbs. very quickly and a few who have dropped over a hundred lbs. over the course of a year. If right now you're even a few lbs. overweight, be honest with yourself and lose the weight. You have everything to gain!

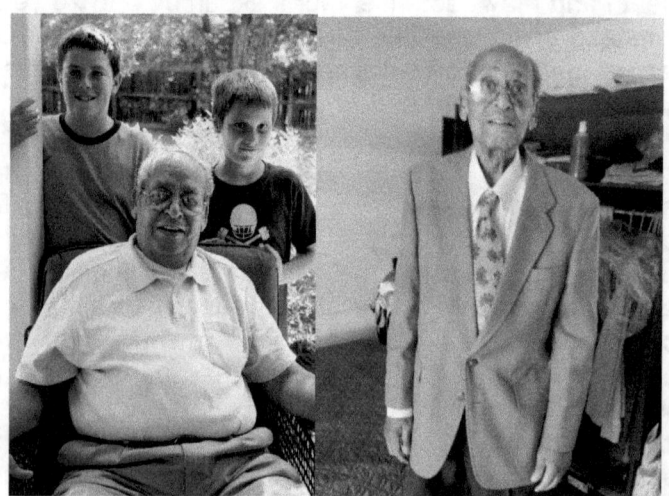

Charles Ellington 'before' & several years 'after'.

ACTION ITEM 16.0
Researchers from Oxford Brookes University in the UK have found measuring a person's height with string, folding that piece of string in half, and making sure that it can fit comfortably around the waist is a better indicator than BMI of whether you have too much body fat. Get some string today and measure yourself!

Chapter 17.
Sweat Much?

Do you ever wonder why some people always seem to be hot or complain they're constantly sweating? Do you fall into this category, or do you have a family member or roommate who complains the thermostat is always set too high? I have a family member and a former roommate who both fall into this category. There are several reasons for this. The first reason should be obvious, but it's not to everyone. If you're more than 10 lbs. overweight, there's a good chance your body will be or will feel warmer than another person's in the same environment who is very skinny. The family member I'm referencing seems to always be hot (even when it's a few degrees below room temperature). She is approximately 20 lbs. overweight and has been for many years. My old roommate Ronald (who wrote the foreword for my first health book: Do These Things or You will Die) was 60 lbs. overweight and often remarked how hot he was. He later admitted to sweating much more years ago before he lost his 60 extra lbs. Even if you're just 10 to 15 lbs. overweight, common sense should indicate that an extra layer of fat around your entire body would insulate your body from cold weather, but at normal room temperatures will make your body feel a lot warmer. The first thing people do before going outside on an extremely cold winter's day is to put on layers. Perhaps you have an undershirt (or thermals), a long sleeve shirt, then a pullover or sweater, an outer jacket, and perhaps a scarf, hat and gloves. Anyone who has gone outside in cold weather (below 32°F), knows how effective the method of layering is to keep your body warm and comfortable (close to the 98.6°F, which is your body's homeostasis). Getting back to Ronald for a minute. When he weighed 225 lbs. on his 5' 9" frame, Ronald essentially had the equivalent of 3 or 4 layers all over his body keeping his body much warmer than myself (I'm 6' and weigh 160 lbs.). No need to dwell on this point anymore and if you still don't understand this simple concept, jump to Action Item # 17 below. Remember the act of sweating (perspiring) is simple: evaporation of sweat from your skin surface has a cooling effect due to the evaporation of water. Hence, in hot weather when your muscles heat up due to exertion, more sweat is produced to keep your body from overheating. The second reason why some people seem to be hot and sweaty more often is due to toxins in their body. When I looked at the diet of my family member I mentioned earlier, it was horrific. She drank coffee, beer, smoked cigarettes, drank Gatorade (much like healthy people guzzle water), and ate a lot of processed foods and a moderate amount of meats. Now even though she tries to eat salads and some healthy foods, if there's enough toxicity in her body, her body when functioning effectively will do anything it can to expel or flush those toxins out of her body. The epidermis (skin) is actually the largest organ in your entire body. One of the fastest and easiest ways to get rid of toxins is by sweating! If you've ever been in a fraternity house early in the morning after a keg party, or have woken up next to anybody who was drinking a lot of alcoholic beverages the night before, you've probably smelled those toxins (alcohol) being expelled through the hung-over person's epidermis. Likewise if you've ever played weekend sports with a group of guys the morning after a night of drinking, you've been around that nasty smell of toxins trying to get evaporated through that person's skin. Many years ago, a few of my fraternity brothers who stuck around Orlando, FL (where we graduated college) started a tradition on Saturday mornings. We enjoyed regular pick-up basketball games across the street from my house. After a few buckets of Hooters' spicy hot chicken wings, several bowls of curly French fries, accompanied by a few pitchers of beer on the Friday night before game day, to say our bodies had an abundance of toxins that needed to be sweated out would be an understatement. A few hours after waking up, we'd all stumble onto the basketball court and one of the toughest (and nastiest) challenges was to guard an opponent on the other team who had both of his arms raised in the air ready to shoot or pass. The smelly armpits from our entire squad was so nasty, that often times in games we'd give the smelly 'shooter' plenty of space to let him take a long range 3-point shot. Anyone who has played pick-up basketball games on a weekend with a bunch of sweaty guys after a night of drinking knows exactly what I'm talking about.... enough said. Now on the other end of the spectrum, I'd been hearing and reading about people on vegan (or vegetarian) diets who never used deodorant. It seemed implausible to me at first. But after much research of the epidermal organ and understanding how the human body eliminates much of its toxicity, this actually makes sense. If someone is vegan and has a very strict diet and eats mostly live plants, vegetables, sprouts, nuts, etc. and very little (if any) alcohol, meats, processed foods, sugar, etc., that healthy person's body doesn't have nearly as much toxicity to expel. Since cleaning my body out for the first time over 10 years ago with the 7-Day "Alkalize & Energize" cleanse (outlined in the appendix of this book), many days I do not use deodorant and I never use anti-perspirant anymore (which actually blocks your sweat glands from doing their natural job). If after detoxifying your body (which I hope everyone reading this book will do) with our 7-Day "Alkalize & Energize" cleanse, and you consider not wanting to use traditional deodorant, feel free to do your own research. Allegedly Cameron Diaz, Bradley Cooper, Matthew McConaughey and several other healthy celebrities (with strict diets) don't use deodorant, or use all-natural deodorant that is healthier than some of the big 'name' brand deodorants and anti-perspirants. Many personal care products that deal with these concerns contain aluminum as an active ingredient, which is a known neurotoxin. This subject has been debated for many years and I'm not going to tackle it here. I'll close by stating that the more toxic food and beverages you consume, the more you will sweat and the nastier you're going to smell!

ACTION ITEM 17.0

Take 3 minutes right now and put on 3 or 4 extra layers of clothes. Add an extra pair of socks, an extra shirt, a pullover, a sweater and a heavy jacket. Put your shoes back on and if you have gloves and a hat, put them on as well. If you're indoors at room temperature, within five minutes notice how your body starts warming up and you might even start sweating. This is an eye-opening exercise and an extra incentive to lose whatever extra weight you may now have!

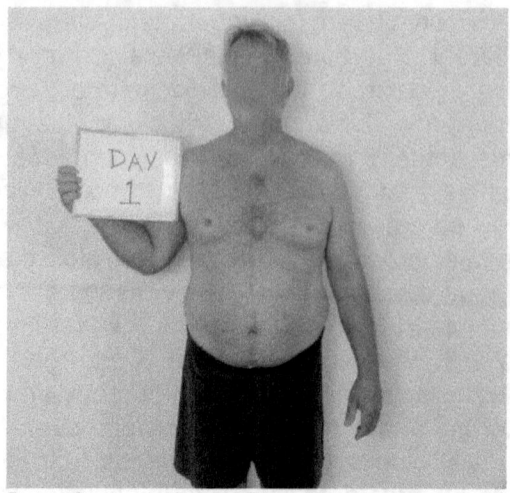

One of my clients on Day 1 having problems
with sweating and wanted to lose weight.

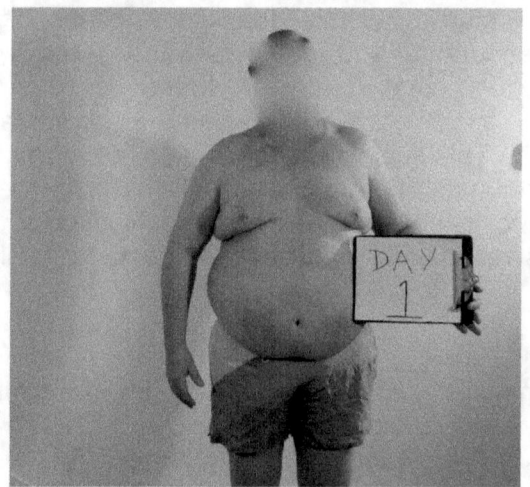

'Local' clients get photographed, weighed in with
witnesses in the studio to document everything.

Chapter 18.
Water: The Essence of Life!

The human body is comprised of almost 70% water. While some people could live for a few weeks without food, water is so critical to the functioning of your brain and other vital organs that most people would die in a matter of days without it. The human brain is almost 80% water and as the central part control center of the nervous system, it coordinates all the functions of the body via electric impulses. The human brain hosts approximately 10 billion neurons (nerve cells)! Without enough water, the nerve network throughout your body would not function properly. Just think about what a great conductor of electricity water is. Water is a vital nutrient to the life of every single cell and (H^2O) is the key component of building these cells. Water regulates your internal body temperature by sweating and respiration. Carbohydrates and proteins that your body uses as food are metabolized and transported by water in the bloodstream. Blood is often called the 'river of life' as it is so essential. Water assists in flushing out toxins, dead cells and other waste mainly through urination and perspiration. Water is the key component of saliva, which is critical in aiding digestion. Water also protects and lubricates joints and serves many other functions critical to life and death. Many employers around the country now post notices, warnings, and even hold educational classes about the dangers of dehydration to keep their workforce healthy and productive. Dehydration, dizziness, heat stroke and other ailments that stem from not drinking enough water can be real health threats. In the film and television industry, the first and most important item producers bring onto every set is plenty of water for the cast and crew. This is such an important matter that Central Casting in Hollywood now mandates everyone who signs up to work in the entertainment business must complete a safety class largely comprised of properly hydrating and avoiding heatstroke. As mentioned in an earlier chapter, when people get tired or feel a lack energy late in the afternoon, a big contributor to this lethargy is a lack of water. I have a large 16 oz. glass of lemon water on my desk as I'm typing this and by habit take a few sips every few minutes to stay hydrated and keep up my energy level. Most people are also tired and groggy when they first wake up. One of the reasons is after many hours of being asleep, their body is water deprived. That's the reason why most people are so thirsty for water first thing in the morning. With every single breath, your lungs expel moisture the same time you're also losing water through your epidermis all night long. Most people don't realize that their brain uses more energy than any other organ in the body. As mentioned, if not properly hydrated your brain (and your entire nervous system) will not conduct electrical energy as efficiently as possible. To get more energy, stay healthy and keep mentally sharp, it is critically important to drink lots of water. Remember alkaline water is preferred as it helps keep your body in a perfectly functioning state of homeostasis. Here are a few specific tips:

1) Drink plenty of pure, clean or filtered (preferably alkaline) water throughout the day.

2) Start drinking water first thing in the morning when you wake up.

3) Soda, milk, juices and other drinks are *not* a substitute for water.

4) Do not drink water (more than a few sips) for at least one hour before going to sleep.

Also a few important warnings: 1) Don't think by drinking alkaline water, that alone will balance your body's pH levels. 2) Make sure most of your diet is from water-rich foods (live vegetables, fruits, sprouts, etc.). 3) Don't drink excessive amounts of alcohol or coffee.

Speaking of water (and specifically water fountains), there's a disturbing trend going on in the U.S. Many schools and universities have ripped out the majority of their water fountains so they can sell more sodas and high-priced beverages. Many businesses have also removed their water fountains and replaced them with vending machines as a revenue source. One large corporation I visited this past year (for an employee health benefits fair) had removed all of their water fountains. Their new Pepsi machines had only one water slot option. I would have bought a bottled Aquafina water for $2.00, but it was sold out! The other vending slots were for Pepsi, Diet Pepsi, Mountain Dew and Slice soda offerings. The entire building had no other drinking water option for over 100 employees! They had even removed the water cooler in the employee break room, as it conflicted with the $2.00 water now being sold. I asked several employees if there was any water source in the building explaining that the vending machine had sold out of water to no avail. I finally discovered a faucet in the kitchen sink, which I used to refill my 16 oz. water bottle multiple times. Looking at this new vending machine model, I'll bet anyone $100 that those employees would drink a lot more *free* water (from a cooler or fountain) than when they have to pay $2.00 per bottle. I'll take the same wager with kids in middle or high school and bet anyone $1,000 that kids would drink more *free* water than when they have to pay $2.00 a bottle. Of course if a 13-year old kid has a choice at the school vending machine between paying for water or getting a Pepsi or Mountain Dew, that kid is most likely going to go for the quick sugar boost and bonus caffeine rush. Later that night when I went through the airport (to fly back to LA), I noticed several of the airport water fountains had been completely removed and in their places were new vending machines selling water and sodas for $5.00! After having just dumped my water out at the TSA screening area two minutes prior, paying $5.00 (even though I get reimbursed by Express Scripts) didn't thrill me, so I searched around the Southwest terminal for 10 minutes and found a water fountain to refill my bottle (a habit I started many years ago). Just like the schools and businesses, it doesn't take a CPA to figure out these vending machines are a very attractive revenue source with millions of travelers streaming through their TSA lines where people are forced to empty all their drinks. But at what cost to people's energy and health?

So how much water should you drink? This is a widely debated topic as there are so many variables. If you're outdoors and running or doing physical labor on a hot day, you'll need to drink more water than someone relaxing inside in the air conditioning. Of course a big factor is how large your body mass is and how much you weigh. I recommend ½ to 1 oz. of water for every lb. of body weight and stay on the high side of that range if you want to be super healthy and hydrated. I weigh 160 lbs. and drink *at least* 160 oz. of water every day. Another rule of thumb I advise is not to drink too much water or flood yourself, but drink just a little bit *more* water than your thirst dictates. By doing this, you err on the side of caution. You'll go to the rest room a bit more often during the day, but that's also a great excuse to get up and step away from your desk for a 2 to 3 minute break, which in itself will give you more energy than if you're sitting motionless at a computer or work station all day. A great water story to share is one about Sarah Smith. Sarah is a 42-year old mother living in the UK. Sarah admitted to not drinking the recommended 2 to 3 liters of water daily. She suffered from poor and sluggish indigestion, experienced regular headaches and joint pains, complained of lack of energy, and had red marks and acne on her skin along with big bags underneath her eyes. She looked 10 years older than her actual age before trying an experiment, which was to drink at least a gallon of water every day for a month. The results were absolutely astounding. In addition to all her ailments going away and feeling increased energy, her skin completely cleared up and she now looks 10 to 15 years younger than before! [18-1]

Another interesting story happened to me last month, which also demonstrates the importance of water consumption to help boost energy levels. I was booked as part of a live studio audience for a new Lifetime Channel reality TV show. I can't share details due to a Non-Disclosure Agreement, but the name of the show is irrelevant. Normally when you're part of a television show or movie that's filming, it's common to work for up to six hours in between the mandated meal breaks. In order to speed up the pace of production and keep the cast, crew and vendors happy, there's usually a large craft service table with plenty of snacks and a large water cooler. In addition to (or in lieu of) the water cooler station, producers usually offer plenty of bottled waters anyone can grab to keep hydrated on set (especially with the heat from all the bright lights). Water bottles are great as they are easy to hide (so they're not seen on camera) and with the cap on if a bottle accidentally tips over, no water is spilled. So this one day I, along with another producer friend, loaded onto the set at 10:00 am and as is my habit, I brought a full water bottle with me to sip on for the next few hours. One of the production assistants came around and made an announcement: "Sorry folks, we start taping in 5 minutes and we can't have any water bottles on set!". A gentleman in front of me politely replied: "That's OK, I'll hide my bottle underneath my chair." That idea didn't go over well with the production team, so the production assistants (three of them) walked around and collected any and all water bottles that many of the 75 audience members had brought to the set. There was a lot of grumbling, but everyone reluctantly turned over their water bottles. This was the first time in 20 years I'd ever seen a live taping where if there was a reasonable place to stash a water bottle, this courtesy was denied. This anti-water plan backfired on the producers later. While a handful of people desperate to use the rest room were allowed the opportunity to sneak off to the rest rooms, the majority of us were seated for a full 6 hours with no food and no water! About 4 hours into the taping, almost all the audience members were slouched over and their energy levels dropping fast. Going into the 5th hour, a few people were literally falling asleep. I only wish I could have snapped a photo of the 75 audience members totally dehydrated (deprived of any water for almost 6 hours) under the hot lights. The 1st Assistant Director (whose job it is to keep the production running and keep on schedule) start calling out individuals and yelling for people to "sit up straight", "smile" and "stop yawning!" Literally almost half of the studio audience members were yawning or nodding their heads right before we broke for our 2:00 pm lunch break. I have to admit, I was one of the many people who was very tired, but it was also a great experiment for me to observe and help prove that drinking water has a major impact on your energy levels. I hope, that if nothing else, this example will encourage you to drink more water and consciously take regular water breaks throughout your day. If you're one of those people who needs a reminder to ease into a new habit, then make yourself a sign or post-it note to put above your desk (or by your computer) that reads: 'Drink More Water!'. There are also several free Android apps now including: 'Drink More Water' and 'Drink Water Beta' and iTunes now offers a 'Water Alarm' app for just $0.99 to help you track your water consumption.

ACTION ITEM 18.0
Make the important decision today to start drinking more water. Make a note to yourself, set an alarm, or download a smartphone app to remind you to start drinking more water to boost your energy and properly hydrate your body. This will be one of the best habits you can instill and will benefit you the rest of your life!

Chapter 19.
"Only the Good Die Young."

As the famous Billy Joel song goes: "Only the Good Die Young". This sad fact seems to be happening more often. A few decades ago, if anyone died young (from my perspective *young* is anyone younger than 50), it would usually be from a car accident or some unusual event. There were a few cases of cancer or diabetes, but they were rare instances and usually these diseases (now epidemic) did not often kill people in their 30's or 40's. The reason I wrote my first health book: Do These Things or You Will Die, was the fact I'd lost over a dozen close friends and family members the last few years to cancer and other terminal diseases including my stepfather, stepbrother, aunts, uncles, and cousins, many of whom were in the prime of their lives. The most shocking losses were my best friend in elementary school, Fritz Collister, my college roommate and fraternity brother, John Clark, and my dear friend and mentor in the film business, Craig Soldinger. Some of these people died in their 30's and 40's. We're now starting to see people get cancer in their 20's! Heart disease is now the # 1 killer in the U.S. and that statistic will soon be overtaken by cancer. Respiratory diseases and diabetes are also growing fast as chronic killers often taking people in the 20's, 30's, or 40's. This growing trend of good people dying young is partially a result of our Standard American Diet (SAD), lack of exercise, and the accepted culture of taking an abundance of pills (either over the counter) or prescription drugs. For me, one way to measure how *healthy* someone is, is to look at whether or not they are taking any prescription drugs, and if so 'how many pills' each day? Below is a table with some startling statistics you won't find in any medical book or research paper. These were from a formal tally I started several years ago and completed during two open enrollment seasons (2014 and 2015) working for Express Scripts for the State of New Mexico retired employees.

DISTURBING TRENDS I RECORDED ON
PRESCRIPTION DRUG USE:

YEAR (S)	TOTAL # OF PEOPLE WHO CAME TO THE EXPRESS SCRIPTS TABLE	# OF PEOPLE I SAW TAKING OVER 20 PRESCRIPTIONS PER DAY!
2005 - 2008	5,985	0
2009 - 2102	6,101	1
2013	5,485	6
2014 - 2015	3,312	7

While giving presentations about their prescription drug changes for the upcoming year, I asked everyone to come to the Express Scripts table afterwards to get information. For the retiree groups (most were over the age of 60), in 2014 approximately 94% were taking some kind of prescription or over the counter drugs on a regular basis. In 2015, approximately 96% were taking daily prescriptions! These statistics were collected from over 2,000 people I spoke to one on one. If I had 100 people stop by my table on a typical day, on average, only 3 to 5 people out of those 100 were not taking any pills! If you don't believe my statistics, think about the following fact released to me by Express Scripts, which I now share in my health benefit fair presentations: "In 2015, there are now over 100,000 different prescription drugs!" This doesn't even count the prescription drugs that are now labeled OTC (over the counter). Chances are if you're over the age of 65 in the U.S., you're taking some sort of prescription drugs every day. So what do the lucky 3 to 5% of "Super Healthy People" I spoke with look like? Some are middle aged and many are in their 70's and 80's. Regardless of their age, these uber-healthy people are usually easy to spot. These 3 to 5% of healthy people are full of energy, have great posture, normally have great looking skin, usually have no ailments, and they're proud of the fact they don't take any pills. This very small, exclusive club of retirees (completely prescription free) started intriguing me about 10 years ago when I started working for Medco (prior to my work at Express Scripts). I started making my own charts to track the very small percentage of retired aged people not taking any prescriptions. At these open enrollment health benefit fairs I worked, almost every person in the audience would stop by my table before or after my presentation (even the non-maintenance drug users), as they would need to get a prescription pricing sheet and/or or get their prescription ID card information for the upcoming year. My table (and the other vendor tables) are usually positioned in the hallway by the entrance to the auditorium (or theater) and I'd count every person who came by. I also asked every one of these 3 to 5 'Super Healthy' people (out of 100) I'd encounter each day: "What's your secret? Please tell me how you are so healthy, and why you've never been on any prescription drugs?". Their answers were almost always the same. As my friend, Tony Robbins says: "Success leaves clues". Do you want to know their secret to successful health? Keep reading and if you too want to be healthy and get off all your prescription drugs, I promise to share these three 'secrets' at the end of the book. By the way, these three secrets (or daily habits) are the same exact three things I tell my clients to do to get healthy, and for those taking any pills - to help get off of their prescription drugs. The amazing results speak for themselves. If you're dying to know these three secrets right now, turn to chapter 36.

ACTION ITEM 19.0
Write down 3 things you think you should be doing to get healthy and hopefully avoid taking any prescription drugs. Think hard about what daily habits unusually healthy people have and you might find the answers.

Chapter 20.
It's Never Too Late. You are What You Eat!

In terms of your diet, *now* is the time to start taking charge of your health. Don't be one of the many people who say: "I'll start my diet tomorrow.", "Next year, I'm going to really start eating better!", "I'm going to focus on my health and eating healthy very soon.", "Come January 1st, look out as I'm starting my healthy diet!" You've probably heard these common excuses before or perhaps you've used one of these excuses yourself. Don't put this important decision off any longer. Even if you think you eat healthy now, why not make a small effort to eat a little bit healthier? There's always room for improvement, and by growing and expanding all areas of our lives, that's what makes our lives better and more interesting. As Charles Ellington proved at 89 years old, "It's never too late to turn your health around" and the best way to begin is by putting better fuel (food) in your body. Did you know that you can get a whole, replacement body (in terms of new cells) every few years? Almost every single cell in the human body is replaced within a seven year period! Some cells are replaced in days, some are replaced in weeks or months, and other cells are replaced over the course of several years. Old cells mature, die off and in their place, brand new cells are formed to eventually replace the old cell. This is exiting news for everyone!

What's even more exciting is how fast you can expel extra acid, toxins, and pesticides out of your body when you change your diet. You truly are what you eat. A good guideline of what foods you should consume are those that are natural, organic (when possible), alkaline and high in water content. In other words, food that grows out of the ground or hangs from a tree vs. something in a box or package. In addition, make sure to drink lots of water every day, since your cells (the building blocks of your body) are mostly water. If you want to jump start this process of replacing and rebuilding healthy, brand new cells, start with the 7-Day "Alkalize & Energize Cleanse". Before you know it, you will become a new you!

ACTION ITEM 20.0

Write down a specific goal on your own or copy this statement below and fill in the blanks: "I will start eating some healthier foods (name 1 or 2 foods) _____
beginning with my commitment to start eating more _____ every day and less _____. I am what I eat!" Post this on your mirror or by your computer screen so you see it every day.

Chapter 21.
Bad Genes?

I can't tell you how many times at health benefits fairs people have walked up to the Medco (or Express Scripts) table after my presentation to ask about their prescriptions and go into a diatribe about how they had "inherited bad genes". I've listened to people talk about their diabetes, high cholesterol, elevated blood pressure, thyroid issues, allergies, obesity, etc. and often times blame it on their bad genes. I'll never forget 10 years ago I was on a cross-country flight to attend an oncology convention (the American Society of Clinical Oncology) and the gentleman in the seat next to me for the 5 ½ hour flight was an oncologist. At this point, I was deep into research about pH balance in the body and the negative effects of acidity and toxicity, while discovering the incredible results of people getting treated by increased alkalinity. I had read about The Gerson Clinic that was turning around the health of hundreds of cancer patients by detoxification, proper nutrition and super alkalizing their systems. I'll let you do your own research on The Gerson Clinic (now operating in Tijuana, Mexico), but I am incredibly impressed how they've received a plethora of patients diagnosed with stage III or stage IV cancer who were sent home to die, and are now perfectly fine decades later! At that time, I was also reading some of Dr. Robert Young's books on alkalinity and was also impressed with the results of his patients at the same time I was incorporating an alkaline lifestyle myself. I became aware of my increased energy levels and the fact that I was never getting sick anymore. I used to get a sinus infection, about once a year, which never happens anymore. Although I might have *off* days now and then where my energy levels are not quite 100% (we all do), I feel so much better and honestly never get sick anymore... not even the flu, which so many people get right after the holidays! So during this lengthy flight (without revealing my background), I decided to delve into a friendly conversation asking this oncologist: "Do you by chance think that improved nutrition and having a more alkaline diet could help minimize the chance of people getting cancer, or possibly improve the odds of beating cancer?" I worded this question carefully so that I would not be in conflict with the standard protocols of oncologists (which in most cases is to recommend an aggressive treatment of chemotherapy, radiation, and/ or surgery). The response the doctor gave me was shocking. He went into a 15-minute explanation that cancer was totally random and had nothing to do with diet or lifestyle, emphasizing that cancer could hit anybody at any time - even people with healthy lifestyles. He claimed nutrition and alkalinity were not factors, stating that the bottom line on people who got cancer was pre-determined by genetics. He said that there was incredible new research going on and they were even getting close to a cure for cancer. This confidant doctor continued that they were making great strides with new chemotherapy drugs (having great success), but the real secret to beating cancer was in new 'Gene Mapping' and understanding DNA sequencing. He boasted that his colleagues were just 2 to 3 years away from figuring out which genes are inherited and how they would soon be able to program and code people's genetic sequences to successfully fight cancer. He concluded his argument by stating: "This is going to be the new future of fighting and beating cancer!" Well, I hate to say it's been a whole decade since that oncologist's grandiose prediction and more people are getting cancer and the success rate of cancer patients surviving and thriving through traditional medicine is abysmal! Whenever I encounter oncologists, traditional medical doctors or cancer patients, I no longer get into an argument or dispute their thinking on traditional cancer treatments... it's a losing battle. I actually understand their logic and thinking, especially when the typical oncologist spends so many years in school studying traditional treatments, the effects of chemotherapy drugs and sometimes decades after that on studies of other cancer patients, peer studies, etc. while maybe getting exposed to preventative medicine and nutrition for a few weeks. I believe that anyone can become an expert in a subject that he or she studies, reads about, and focuses on for many years. That oncologist I spoke to was clearly a cancer expert and I respect that. However my focus (and one of my missions in life now) is to enlighten and educate people about how tens of thousands of people (who supposedly had 'bad genes') through diet, lifestyle changes and in some cases non-conventional treatments and therapies now live healthy, normal lives decades after they were diagnosed with terminal cancer! One of the most important things I stress to friends who get diagnosed with cancer is instead of worrying and thinking about all the people who didn't survive, think about the many people who have overcome cancer. There are hundreds of household names who have beaten cancer you've probably heard of who can inspire your journey including: Suzanne Somers, Hugh Jackman, Mark Ruffalo, Christina Applegate, Edie Falco, Lance Armstrong, Drew 'Dr. Drew' Pinsky, Tom Green, Laurence 'Mr. T.' Tureaud, Sheryl Crow, Kathy Bates, Sharon Osbourne, Rod Stewart, and many others. All of these people (after their life altering 'wake-up calls') have improved their lifestyles to put the odds in their favor that they will not have a cancer recurrence. So here are my beliefs on what causes cancer and what role your genes play. I firmly believe that your lifestyle including many factors like your diet, daily exercise patterns, other environmental factors (like the quality of the air you breathe and water your drink), and your overall daily thoughts (your daily attitude and outlook on life) probably account for 90% of your cancer risk. I also believe that people's genetics are a small factor (perhaps 10% of your risk). If there is a history in your family of leukemia, Addison's disease, hemophilia, etc. those are real risks that can be passed down genetically. Most of the common diseases or ailments today including Type II diabetes, heart disease, most cancers, COPD, etc. are induced by lifestyle choices and are absolutely reversible! Below are five pieces of science based evidence to back up my theory that in most cases, lifestyle decisions affect your health, instead of the 'bad genes' that the media and medical community often hype as the culprit:

1) The current obesity trend in America vs. other countries with different lifestyles. "69% of adults are either overweight or obese", reports CBS Atlanta. "The average American was 33 pounds heavier than a Frenchman, 40 pounds heavier than a citizen of Japan, and 70 pounds heavier than a person in Bangladesh." [21-1] Since the population in American has become more diverse in the last 30 years than ever before (in terms of different nationalities and ethnic backgrounds), that nullifies the genetic argument.

2) <u>The China Study</u>. A comprehensive book, which examines the relationship between the consumption of animal products (including dairy) and chronic illnesses such as coronary heart disease, diabetes, and all types of cancer. It was the most comprehensive study on nutrition ever. Research was done on thousands of people (it spanned across 65 different counties in China) and included family groups and some twins (to help look at genetic factors). The most startling fact revealed was in certain counties where the Chinese population started consuming meat, the incidents of cancer increased 400%! If you study Dr. T. Colin Campbell's work (Dr. Campbell was one of the authors of the study), he also found that casein (the protein in cow's milk) literally triggers the cancer gene. That's one of the reasons why developed countries like the U.S. and the U.K. are losing the breast cancer battle (and most other cancer battles), while countries like Bhutan and Gambia (with a plant based diet) see very few breast cancer cases. [21-2]

3) Studies done on multiple generations of Japanese who moved to the U.S. clearly demonstrate each successive generation in the U.S. are more obese and have developed more health problems than those family members who stayed in Japan. [21-3] Once again, this is more evidence that diet and lifestyle seem to be more important than genetics.

4) The same effect has been happening in China recently (during the last 20 years). Obesity is skyrocketing along with many of the western culture diseases such as Type II diabetes, heart disease and cancer. [21-4] Western fast-food restaurants are rapidly expanding all over China and soda is replacing water and tea as the favorite beverage. Meat and dairy are replacing the traditional food staples of vegetables and rice. At the same time, millions of Chinese are replacing their bicycles for cars as the country keep shifting away from farming towards factories and manufacturing. You can read about this Chinese phenomenon on almost any news outlet. Once again, these populations have similar genes, but it is the radically changing lifestyles that have transformed the health of the current generation in less than two decades.

5) The many studies done on the entire population of Norway between 1940 to 1945 during the peak of World War II. Heart disease alone plummeted over 50%! Look once again at the chart at the end of chapter 5 if you need to refresh your memory.

It's been said in the medical community that some people's DNA might carry a genetic code making them slightly more susceptible to certain health conditions or diseases. However, with so much new evidence (showing tens of thousands of cases) where people have overcome cancer or actually reversed a disease or medical condition from lifestyle changes, why wouldn't you want to dramatically improve your odds of a happy, healthy life? In conclusion, here's a great quote from Dr. Colin Campbell who's been studying this issue for decades: "Population studies begun forty to fifty years ago show that when people migrate from one country to another, they acquire the cancer rate of the country to which they move, despite the fact their genes remain the same." It is pretty tough to argue with that!

ACTION ITEM 21.0
Do your own research today to find one example of how lifestyle is more important than genetics in terms of most diseases and cancer.

<u>SECTION II: MOVE!</u>

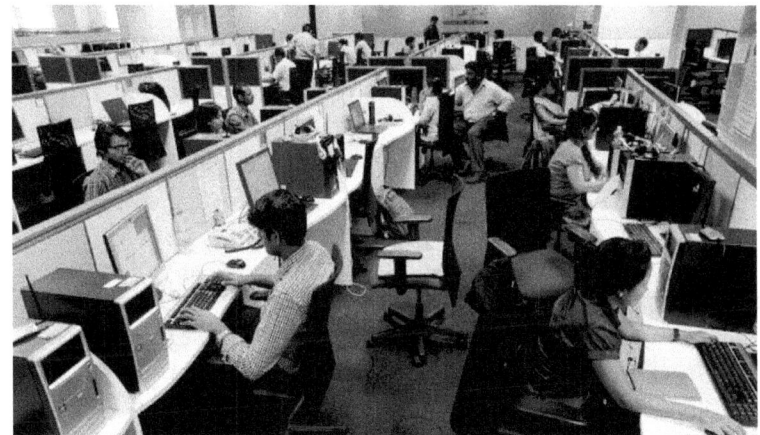

Today's office environments do
not promote a lot of body movement.

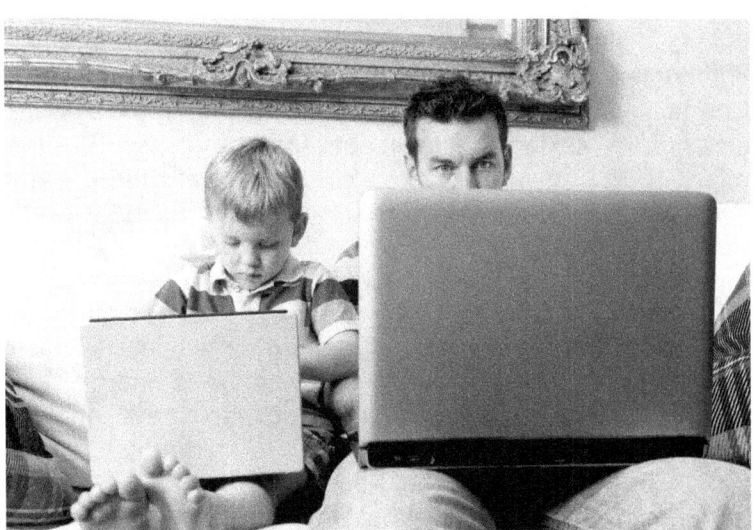

Neither do most modern family activities.

Chapter 22.
Even if You Don't Work Out;
This Must be a Priority!

Let's be honest, not everyone likes working out. I don't always like the thought of going to my gym on a gorgeous California day to lift a bunch of heavy weights. Just the words 'working out' don't seem very appealing after a long, hard day at work. I do, however, go to the gym a few times a month, because I feel amazing afterward. So if you're not a gym rat and don't enjoy going to the gym multiple times a week that's fine. You don't need to worry. You don't even have to go 'work out' in a gym anywhere, but you do need to move your body! Furthermore, you must decide unequivocally that your health is a priority. In addition to fueling your body with the proper, all-natural foods covered in the earlier chapters of the book, you must prioritize moving your body every single day with no exceptions! Sometimes at my live events, I'll start the program off writing on a large white easel pad and ask the audience to list out the top priorities in their lives. What priorities or things are most important to them? The audience will often shout out: "family", "faith", "career", "happiness", "close friends", "finances", etc. Ironically *health* is not the first priority that is shouted out (even at a 'Health' event)! Normally health is the third or forth item on people's lists. I continue by asking the audience and sometimes I'll even offer $100 to anyone who can challenge me if there's any item on their list that doesn't depend on health first? People in the audience usually quiet down and eventually agree that every single aspect of their lives depends upon their health first. Most successful business people and leaders need vibrant health and energy to achieve all their lofty goals and plans. You can't give time and energy back to your family and loved ones if you don't have enough energy at the end of the day. It's hard to start a new project or hobby, after a full day at work if you don't have vibrant health and energy! Once you figure this out, I hope that right now (as you're reading this) that you will make your health (and moving your body) the # 1 priority in your life! This has to be a *must* for you, rather than just a *should*. I can't overstate the importance of moving your body on a daily basis. I make exercising first thing in the morning (as soon as I hop out of bed at 4:30am) a *must* for several reasons: 1) In just a few minutes, I wake up my entire body and start feeling better. 2) By getting my blood flowing faster and more oxygen circulating, my entire metabolism is jump started. 3) My energy and mental clarity get a huge boost before I start my day. 4) This automatically triggers my Lymphatic System (more on this in chapter 27). As mentioned above, you don't have to go the gym. Right in your own home, you can do a few quick push ups, sit ups, stretches, yoga, resistance floor exercises, rubber band exercises, jumping jacks, or go outside for a brisk 20 minute walk, etc. Once you instill this daily habit and find out how great you feel, you'll be addicted to this. One of my good friends, Alexandra Paul, sums it up best:

> "Sometimes I wake up in the morning and go ahh...
> I don't want to work out! But I do anyway, because
> I'll always feel better afterwards. I have never once
> worked out and felt worse."

People who visit Hollywood remark that many of the people who live here seem to be leaner and in great shape. I don't like to generalize, but after living in L.A. for many years, I've also noticed the majority of the local population seem to be in pretty good health and I don't notice as many obese people as I see in some of the southeastern states. There are a few reasons why I think this is true:

1) People in the entertainment business have an extra incentive to be in great shape if they're in front of the camera, or being interviewed (it's true that "the camera adds 15 lbs.").

2) The weather is great all year round, which makes it easier to exercise every day.

3) Hollywood is surrounded by hills, forests, mountains, and the ocean making activities like hiking, biking, surfing, swimming, skiing, etc. accessible to just about everyone.

4) There seems to be more fitness and health clubs, yoga studios, etc. here than in any other city I've been to.

5) Peer pressure - if your family, friends, co-workers, neighbors, etc. have healthy habits, that tends to influence and rub off on you. On that last note, there have been multiple studies that show: "Obese parents increase kids' risk of being overweight." [22-1] Bad habits of not exercising, or not eating healthy can rub off not only within peer groups, but especially in the same household when children look to their parents as role models.

In addition to *moving your body* first thing in the morning, you can also easily *move your body* during the day even if you have a super busy work schedule like many people do. I'll go into great detail about the exciting concept of how to exercise in 'No Extra Time' in chapter 28.

ACTION ITEM 22.0
Decide right now (this very moment) that you will make moving your body every day your # 1 priority. Set a goal that you will do this for at least seven (7) days. Once you do, I'm confident you'll continue this daily habit as you notice how you start feeling better and have more energy!

Chapter 23.
How Old is 'Old'?

You've probably heard the expression: "Age is a state of mind". I believe that's truer now than ever before. The U.S. has a longer life expectancy than previous decades (now in the upper 70's), but as a general population we're more obese, on more drugs, and sicker than previous generations. I have friends in their 80's and 90's who are amazingly fit and active, who can run circles around people in their 60's. On the contrary, have you ever seen anyone in their 50's (perhaps overweight, not very active, on prescription drugs with a few ailments) who look like they are in their 60's or 70's?

Nobody should think that life is winding down or start placing physical restrictions on themselves in their 50's or 60's, especially if they take care of their bodies. In fact, Robbins Research International reviewed studies from different Universities that showed people in their 60's have been able to get the same muscle function and capacity as people in their 20's and 30's! [23-1] Part of these results are from good nutrition and from a positive mind set, but a big part of these results is a specific type of training called Static Contraction Training (SCT), which I've been doing myself for years, and which Tony Robbins and many professional athletes endorse. Even if you don't do any specific type of work out, there is always hope based upon your life style. Many years ago when traveling through the small villages of northern Thailand up in the hills near Chang Mai, I noticed older men lugging around lumber, heavy water buckets, and other supplies. Nobody forced these men (or women) to retire at 65 and certainly none of their peers encouraged them to get a lazy boy recliner and park their butt in front of a television set for most of their days. These men I saw (estimated to be in their 70's and 80's) were walking 10 to 12 miles between villages and remained very active every single day! As mentioned before, I have many friends here in the U.S. in their 80's and 90's who are extremely fit, healthy and energetic. My father didn't retire until he was 82 and he can probably out speed-walk a percentage of people 20 years younger than him, simply because he walks consistently every day and works out with a trainer several days each week. Below are some other examples of people who are not going to let the number of candles on their birthday cake slow them down:

- While hiking the Santa Monica mountains one weekend, I ran into the 'Over the Hill Gang'. They are a hiking club in the L.A. area made up of retirees (including some in their 80's and 90's) who get together to hike, bike, kayak, go running, etc. every weekend.

- Last weekend I was riding around the San Fernando Valley and pulled up to a stop light next to two very fit ladies (ages 85 and 72) who were out for a 45-mile bike ride around the valley.

- Harriet Thompson is a 92-year-old Marathon runner from Charlotte, NC who still goes the full 26 miles and finishes most of her races in well under 8 hours.

- Poland's Stanislaw Kowalski is one the world's oldest athletes still competing at 105. He competes in the 100-meter race, completing it most recently in just 34.50 seconds. That's a lot faster than some friends I know who are 40 years younger!

Whenever someone tells you to "stop acting like a kid and act your own age", "slow down", or "hang up the skis", don't listen to them. Find a new peer group (like the 'Over the Hill Gang') or look for some new references of people your age who are looking to climb Mount Everest, run a marathon, go skydiving, go white water rafting, or some other adventure. Don't let anybody tell you that turning 70, 80 or 90 is 'old'. They are just numbers. How you take care of and maintain your body, and how you choose to pursue your passions in life are what really counts. A video very apropos to this chapter was shared with me this morning. It showed Virginia McLaurin, a small lady with big energy walking into the White House to meet President Obama. When Virginia walked in and saw the President for the first time, she shouted out, smiled and literally started dancing she was so thrilled! After their dancing celebration President Obama asked Ms. McLaurin: "What's the secret to still dancing at 106?" Virginia immediately replied back: "Just keep moving!"

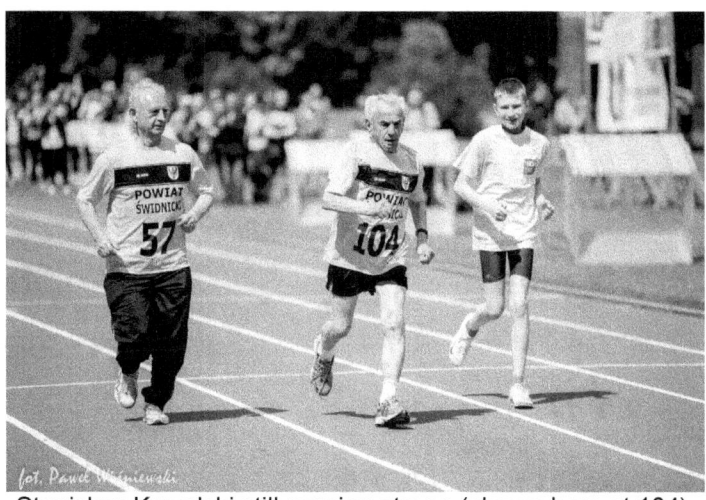

Stanislaw Kowalski still running strong (shown here at 104).

ACTION ITEM 23.0

Do an internet search for 1 or 2 people your age who still compete in athletic competitions, travel the world, or pursue their passions like someone much younger. This will give you a completely new perspective truly on how old is 'old'?

Chapter 24.
Sitting Yourself to Death

In the U.S., the average number of years men get to enjoy in retirement is only 10 years.[24-1] A study reported by Tony Robbins (from Robbins Research Institute), revealed that the most men in the U.S. die within 3 years of retiring! This holds true for men who go from working full time straight to retirement. For women it's a few years longer, but think about this shocking statistic for a moment... this means after all those years studying in school, and then another 40 to 50 years working at a job (that many people in the U.S. don't truly love), statistically they won't even get to enjoy 10 years of retirement before they're dead! There are a few reasons for this, one of which is the lack of routine and 'purpose' in retired people's lives, but the main reason I believe is that many people in this country retire to their favorite lounge chair or sofa in front of the 'Boob Tube'. Not only does excessive sitting shave years off your lifespan, but sitting for long periods of time precludes lack of movement, which in itself saps your energy. Over time retired people tend to spend more time in their chair or couch with less movement until there's no movement at all. No movement at all of course is death! All medical doctors and health experts agree that daily body movement adds years to your life, while remaining sedentary shortens one's life span. A new study presented at the European Society of Cardiology (ESC) Congress suggests that regular exercise increases one's life span and that just 25 minutes of brisk walking a day can add up to 7 years to your life! [24-2] The decline when people fully retire and become sedentary can become a slow death spiral. Without a daily exercise routine, sport, or a long daily walk, people notice a decline in energy. Over time, your body will start to atrophy and you have even less energy. After all, that big chair is so inviting and comfortable isn't it? The double whammy of spending retirement in a lounger is that in addition to the lack of movement and boredom is often accompanied by snacking. It's pretty easy while you're plopped down on the couch watching your favorite TV show to snack on some popcorn or enjoy a big bowl of ice cream. Perhaps you enjoy a few sodas or a few cold beers? After all, you've worked your whole life for your retirement... shouldn't you get to enjoy it? This vicious cycle continues over a few years until the retired victim needs a scooter, a walker, or a cane to get around. Ultimately that same sedentary person may need in-home care or have to go to a nursing home for assistance getting up out of their chair and into bed. Once again, the difference between life and death is movement! After seeing many healthy people in their 90's (and a few over 100) walking and hiking on trails around California, there's no reason for people in their 60's or 70's to die so soon after their retirement! About eight years ago I visited Denmark for a diabetes conference on behalf of Novo Nordisk and I wondered why Danish people had a much lower diabetes rate than the rest of the European countries. I was also curious why Danish people appeared to be so healthy and fit. At that point a few private employers in Copenhagen were experimenting with 'standing desks', which I'm afraid to admit I had never heard of. In Denmark, employers are now required by law to provide their employees with adjustable desks so they can stand if they choose. [24-3] Can you imagine how many millions of people we could help in the U.S. if we got them up off their butts? It would be similar to 100 years ago when the majority of America's workforce was actually standing and obesity and all the accompanying diseases were very rare. To purchase standing desks would be an upfront investment by private companies and the government, but it would also save billions in long-term health care and dramatically boost productivity! If you start searching for standing desks, it can be expensive (some cost over $1,000). While you can't put a price on your health, there is one company I've discovered that has a great product for a reasonable price. Check out: www.attollodesk.com. Another temporary option (if you're tight on money but want the benefits of standing right away) is a DIY standing desk. 'Do it Yourself' by getting a large plastic tub or laundry basket and on top of that, place an appropriate sized smooth plywood board or glass plate as your desk surface. Simply measure the desktop area you'd like and most hardware stores will cut the wood or glass to your desired size for free. I got so inspired, that I initially went this route and for less than $15, I made my own standing desk in about an hour! My perfectly elevated desk area (my desktop is smooth plywood) is large enough to hold my laptop, mouse pad and mouse, cell phone, alkaline water, etc. By the way, another side benefit of utilizing a standing desk is you normally will have much better posture. This habit in itself if great for sore backs and boosts your energy! Ask any chiropractor about standing tall and they will all agree, it's one of the best ways to fix bad posture and back problems. One other really cool product I recommend is the 'Wurf Board'. It is proven science that compares *static standing* (like most of us do when we actually stand) vs. *active standing* (which helps your balance and burns calories while having fun)! Think of it like surfing at your standing desk or simply use the Wurf Board on it's own. Check out www.Wurf.com. If you still don't believe what a problem sitting is for your health, do your own research. There are now hundreds of studies confirming the link between excessive sitting and premature death. One recent study, from the Pennington Biomedical Research Center in Baton Rouge, LA followed 17,000 Canadians over 12 years and found that those who sat for most of the day were 54% more likely to die of heart attacks than those who didn't. [24-4] Remember that the American Medical Association (AMA) has now officially recognized obesity as a disease. All the new findings from excessive sitting are spawning a new diagnosis called 'Sitting Disease'. In my opinion, you have two choices: 1) Start taking drugs for all these so-called 'new' diseases or 2) Stand Up For Your Health. I choose to stand up and feel amazing!

ACTION ITEM 24.0

Do an honest assessment of how much time you sit each day. Make it a point to stand up and take a break at least once an hour. If you have a desk job, look into purchasing a standing desk or ask your employer if they can subsidize a standing desk. Or you can build your own raised desk as described above.

Chapter 25.
Posture: Very Important, but Neglected

Humans were designed to stand tall and upright and sleep on a flat, hard surface. That's why standing desks and firm mattresses are recommended. People were never meant to sit in cheaply designed office chairs with their shoulders and arms hunched over a desk typing or checking e-mails eight hours a day. Ask any chiropractor what the biggest problem is with their patients and they'll tell you: "It used to be people working at their computers while falling into bad posture habits". Over time, this poor posture creates real problems for your joints including the back, shoulders, neck, arms, hips, etc. Just like the problem of carpal tunnel syndrome (which has become a big problem over the last 20 years), one of the biggest NEW problems today which didn't exist 5 years ago is often referred to as 'text neck'. Human necks were never designed to be hunched over with our heads looking straight down at a smart phone in an unnatural position. Yet in this modern world, too many of us spend our days with our heads slumped over for a simple reason: we're staring at the tiny screen of a smartphone or tablet. People spend an average of 2 to 4 hours each day with their necks bent over in this unnatural angle while shooting off emails or responding to texts. That's 700 to 1,400 hours a year in this unnatural position! [25-1] Common sense should dictate that forcing our bodies (and our joints) into completely unnatural and sometimes uncomfortable positions for hours at a time will create problems. The trap we all fall into (including myself from time to time) is that it's so easy to slump, slouch or look down at our computer or smartphone screens, unless we make a concentrated effort to change that. Here are two helpful tips that have helped me enormously over the past few years: 1) Put a Post-it note or tape a message near your computer screen to 'CHECK POSTURE' where you'll see it often and be reminded. 2) If you already have the excellent habit of drinking lots of water all day, you'll automatically be getting up for regular restroom breaks. You can also set a timer on your watch or smartphone to get up and walk around every hour for a few minutes. Those two tips have kept me much more aware of my posture and minimize the possibility that my joints get fixed in an unnatural position for a long of a time. An additional tip I suggest to avoid text neck, is to learn to text less, use Siri, or at least be aware of your head and neck posture, so that you can take breaks or minimize the poor texting posture. If you do these things, you'll have more energy, feel better, and will be much less likely to see a chiropractor. Remember that proper posture is very important for your health and productivity, so don't neglect it!

ACTION ITEM 25.0
Stand in front of a mirror or turn on and reverse the camera on your phone to analyze your posture. Are your shoulders back and level? Is your head up with your ears over your shoulders? Are you standing tall with a slight, natural bend in the knees? Observe your posture and if needed, implement some of the tips shared above, especially if you sit at work all day.

Chapter 26.
"Take it Easy…"

One of the most famous songs in history is by the Eagles and titled: "Take It Easy". Listen to this song if you haven't heard it in a while and learn not to push yourself too hard. This doesn't mean to not have drive, passion, or set extremely lofty goals. Just don't push yourself too hard all the time. Take it easy now and then to allow your body and mind to rest and also for you to enjoy more of life! Not pushing yourself too hard all the time is a very important tip for your overall health for several reasons. This chapter will alert and warn you about the two examples where many people 'push too hard' and jeopardize their health: 1) The first example is when 'Type-A' personalities or hard-charging business people lose balance in their lives and simply push themselves too far - often towards a heart attack! You've probably witnessed someone trying to meet a deadline (working 20+ hour days and taking a 3 to 4 hour nap), or the workaholic who works 10 to 12 hour days and brings his or her work home with them for another few hours. I've seen people pushing so hard that they continue to type on their laptop and talk on their smart phones during their 10-minute lunch break while they're frantically trying to force food down their throats with veins bulging out of their neck. Long term, this lifestyle of working too many hours and not getting enough sleep will not only ruin your relationships with family and friends, but it may well lead to a heart attack! In the event that you don't suffer a heart attack, this constant stress of overworking, lack of sleep and often combined with too much coffee or other stimulants will break down your immune system and can lead to high blood pressure, severe stress, disease and/or cancer. I saw this happen to one family member and several friends who are no longer with us today, but rather buried six feet under the ground. Remember that stress (especially extreme or long term stress) creates acid in your body and the damage over time can be fatal. 2) The second example is when people push themselves too hard during exercise. This advice would not necessarily apply to an Olympic or world-class athlete preparing for a major sporting event (who has proper supervision, coaches, trainers, and nutritionists). This example is for the rest of us mortals who exercise to keep in shape, play weekend sports, etc. There is a long-standing, protective defense mechanism in our bodies, which stimulates lactic acid when we push our muscles too far for too long. If you've ever attempted pull-ups or done curls with heavy weights, after a few reps your biceps start burning and can actually start hurting. This is from a build up of lactic acid in that specific muscle area, so that you stop doing those curls before you damage your muscles. If you're a gym rat who over trains and does not give your muscles a proper rest, recovery and re-growth period, this can sometimes be counter productive. When I have clients (especially those with cancer), I tell them when doing the 7-Day "Alkalize & Energize" cleanse, to not do anything strenuous that would stimulate the production of lactic acid. The last thing a stage III or stage IV cancer patient needs is more acid being dumped into their body! One of my early clients Ronald Farnham, (we worked together closely for about a year) was trying to lose body fat and trim down before his next baseball season started. The few times Ronald purposely went against my advice when I told him no strenuous exercise, he got interesting results. During a few days on one of his cleanses when he chose to do wind sprints and was practicing his pitching at full speed, he did not lose any weight despite exerting those extra calories. If you need to, go back and re-read chapter 11 on Alkalinity. This is an extremely important concept for anyone wanting to get in shape or lose a few extra pounds. I explain why so often people who work out too hard cannot lose the last few pounds they're trying to lose, due to the stimulation of lactic acid (which in turn signals the body to store more fat to protect their internal organs from that extra acid). This acid creation - fat storage vicious cycle will go on forever if you keep pushing yourself too hard. That's why so many of my clients for the first time in their life easily lose 7 to 15 pounds in their first seven days. You can be like my old, stubborn self many years ago who would push myself like crazy in all kinds of sports and also go to the gym 4 to 5 days a week, or you can take it easy. When I was in my 20's and 30's, I wanted to chisel my body, so I could least have 'six-pack' abs like I saw on the cover of Men's Fitness magazine. Instead all I ever got were slightly bigger muscles and continued 'love handles' that I could never,

ever get rid of. Once I decided to take it easy, by not pushing myself so hard in the gym (in fact I don't even go to the gym while I do the 7-Day "Alkalize & Energize" cleanse), I got rid of my love handles for the very first time in my life and even saw a six-pack where my well rounded stomach used to protrude! Ask any personal trainer and they will admit that shaping your body isn't done alone in the gym, it mostly takes place in the kitchen. To me that whole idea tastes a lot better and seems a lot easier! One last thought to share is from longevity expert Aubrey de Grey. In his studies, he made this discovery you may have heard before: "When you look at people around the world who live past 100, the one thing they all share in common is a laid back happy attitude." Another reminder to all of us who want to stay healthy and happy into our triple digit years. Just take it easy...

ACTION ITEM 26.0

If you're running yourself ragged (at work or at home), take a breath and write down at least one bad habit that you're going to stop for at least one week. Perhaps you're working too many hours, staying up late, or working out too often and not giving your body a chance to rest and recover. Choose one of these bad habits and for at least one week, just take it easy!

Chapter 27.
Who Takes Out Your Trash?
The Lymphatic System

One of your body's most important functions that few people (including medical doctors) ever talk about is a healthy lymphatic system, which essentially 'takes out your body's trash'. The removal of dead cells, excess acids and proteins, toxins, potential poisons and anything harmful to your well-being is the job of your lymphatic system. A healthy lymphatic system can be a matter of life and death! What's most shocking is that many oncologists don't sit down with their cancer patients and explain the importance of the lymphatic system to help remove toxins along with the large amounts of potentially harmful chemicals during and after chemotherapy. I know because I've spoken to several cancer patients and also attended many oncology conferences and 99% of the discussions are on the new treatment protocols. Most people know about the pulmonary system's pump: the lungs; the circulatory system's pump: the heart; but don't realize the lymphatic system (one of your body's most critical) has no pump! Here is Merriam-Webster's definition of lymph: "a usually clear coagulable fluid that passes from intercellular spaces of body tissue into the lymphatic vessels, is discharged into the blood by way of the thoracic duct and right lymphatic duct, and resembles blood plasma in containing white blood cells and especially lymphocytes". [27-1] This lymph is basically the waste fluid and excess protein that has been squeezed out of the blood and drained from the tissue in microscopic blind-ended vessels called lymph capillaries to the thousands of lymph nodes. These lymph nodes filter the lymphatic fluids, which contain white blood cells that attack and kill any infectious microorganisms and help remove toxins, poisons, etc. This YouTube video below by www.BalancedHealthToday.com explains more:

http://www.youtube.com/watch?v=XtkrN2hnK-o.

There are two critically important messages to take away about your lymphatic system: 1) The more processed, toxic, acidic foods and drinks (trash) you allow into your body, the harder it is on your digestive system and also your lymphatic system. 2) The lymphatic system runs down a one-way street draining lymph from the tissue and returning it to the blood without a central pump. To facilitate the draining of this lymph, you need to do exercise, which activates muscle stimulation and/or do deep diaphragmic breathing, which stimulates your lymphatic system like a vacuum or pump. These two points are reinforced by the fact that exercise makes you feel energized immediately and the interesting trivia fact that athletes on the average are seven times less likely to get cancer! The lymphatic system is often compared to a city's sanitation service filtering out waste products, toxins, poisons and any material that could cause infections, disease or cancer. With modern day processed food and the massive quantities of meats, pastas, sodas, sugars, etc. we now consume in the U.S., it's no surprise that our lymphatic systems (our sanitation systems) are overtaxed. To make matters worse, most people in sedentary office jobs get distracted and don't make a priority of moving every hour, so they often feel fatigued. If you start doing any kind of exercise on a daily basis (walking, running, cycling, hiking, lifting weights, tennis, etc.) you will feel more energized. Here's a great visual: instead of minimizing your trash by conservation, recycling, etc. and then putting this actual household trash into nice neat garbage bags at the end of your driveway so that the garbage man can easily pick it up every few days, imagine creating an excess amount of trash and simply throwing this trash all over your front yard. First of all, your trash will start leaking household toxins (including today's cleaning products, bleaches, insecticides) that will start killing your lawn, and secondly your garbage man is going to be overwhelmed! If enough trash piles up in your yard and this goes on long enough, you'll start having insects, rats and other rodents come out until your yard becomes a waste hazard. In a way, this is what many people are doing to their own bodies. Many of us eat too much processed or acidic food which piles up in our intestines and colon and over time this putrefied food decays inside our bodies creating major problems like too much acid (which leads to ulcers), or excess stress on certain organs like our liver, stomach, intestines, colon, etc. When people eat excess amounts of acidic, processed food and don't exercise or breathe properly (to stimulate their lymphatic system) this can lead to all kinds of disease, cancer, etc. Another potential danger of your lymphatic system not working properly is gout or edema, which is a swelling in part of your body (often your legs, arms, or even fingers) where excess lymph fluid is not disposed of properly. This is a serious problem and you should see a doctor immediately! This problem is often seen with sedentary or older people who have a bad diet and limited exercise. When their health really declines, they often end up in a wheelchair, which makes their bodies even more immobile, and can lead them into a downward health spiral. The good news is that there are two *easy* ways to immediately trigger your lymphatic system! 1) Rapid body movement - any kind of exercise like lifting weights or active sports are great, but if you're not a 'work out' type of person, that's OK... just take a fast walk for at least 15 minutes and get your body moving. This will get your blood pumping and your lymphatic system flowing. A great tip (and you often see speed walkers doing this) is to also swing your arms while you're walking. The more body movement the better. For people who live in extreme temperature environments where walking outside in a winter blizzard is not a safe option, try getting a small rebounder trampoline. A small trampoline can stow underneath your bed or in your closet and you can bounce for 10 to 15 minutes every morning. Start very slow and easy if you're not in great shape. Take a few small easy bounces for just a few minutes, work up to 5 minutes, and eventually your goal over time should be to bounce for at least 15 minutes every morning. 2) Deep diaphragmic breathing - as soon as I finish writing this chapter this morning, I'm going outside for my 20 minute 'walk and jog'. For the first 10 minutes (before jogging), I speed walk and concentrate on talking long, deep breaths (I inhale through my nose for 5 seconds, hold that breath for 10 seconds, and slowly exhale through my mouth for 7 seconds). When breathing in, stand tall and keep your body posture straight, taking deep breaths through your belly, while at the same time allowing your lungs to expand to their maximum capacity. If you can't do a 5, 10, 7 count initially, that's OK. Start with a smaller, easier breath pattern that's more comfortable for you. Over time you will build up your lung's capacity and your breathing pattern will get deeper and longer which will stimulate your lymphatic system! Following up on the importance of breathing, yoga is one of the best exercises in the world and known for its focus on deep breathing. If you've never tried yoga before, don't take my word for it, ask a friend or family member. There are literally too many positive health benefits of yoga to list here. There are yoga classes for people of all ages and levels from the beginner to the most advanced. I have to give a shout out to my friend Diamond Dallas Page as he has literally invented or created (after suffering a career debilitating injury where he couldn't even walk) an incredible, unique yoga program called DDP Yoga. Check out his website: www.DDPYoga.com or anyone in the Los Angeles area can check out his programs in person. Dallas also has great DVDs and a mobile app to do his DDP Yoga anywhere. For anyone else outside of LA and having trouble finding a general yoga class (that also fits into your budget), check out www.YogaAnytime.com and www.YogaGlow.com. If Swami Sivananda can make time for breathing exercises and do yoga every day at 120 years old, so can you (that '120' was *not* a typo by the way). There's no longer any excuse for not filling your lungs with fresh air, getting your blood circulating and stimulating your lymphatic system for peak performance and on your way towards better health!

ACTION ITEM 27.0

Decide on one of the options above to stimulate your lymphatic system today! If you don't have time for dedicated exercise (like yoga), you should start with at least doing 10 to 15 minutes of deep, diaphragmic breathing. Whichever option you choose, you'll immediately feel a boost of energy when you're done. The more you move your body and/or do these breathing exercises, the better you'll feel!

Chapter 28.
No Time to Exercise? Try 'NET' Time!

NET is an acronym that stands for 'No Extra Time' and I heard about this profound concept many years ago from Tony Robbins. Tony mentioned how he used this principle to run his personal life (being married with several kids), manage his seven different companies, keep up with his speaking engagements all over the world (on the road almost 300 days per year!), and still enjoy his hobbies like flying, and maintain his incredible energy and health! Tony's concept really works and in my last book I shared how you too can use this powerful 'NET' principle to manage your busy schedule while keeping health a top priority. All legitimate health experts and medical doctors agree that exercise is a critical part of good health. There's no way around this golden rule. It doesn't mean you have to go to the gym three days a week, be part of a Cross-Fit program, or run 30 miles every weekend. However, the key is you have to keep your body moving every day. Even if you're not an 'exercise buff', I hope you'll read this chapter and implement some of the strategies of NET time. There are dozens of reasons why people don't go to the gym, go running, bicycling, hiking, play sports, work outdoors in the garden, etc., but the most common excuse I hear: "I just don't have time". In our busy, modern lives, time is the most precious commodity, so there is some validity to this excuse, but if you understand this concept of multi-tasking or doing several things (including exercise) at the same time, you'll be able to get exercise in 'No Extra Time'! A great example of this is an uber-efficient businessman and friend of mine named Tom who has an hour-long commute every morning. Instead of just driving and listening to talk radio and letting obnoxious drivers influence his state every morning, Tom (an agent in Beverly Hills) utilizes NET time by making a short list of three or four important clients on the east coast he needs to speak with. While it's 8:00 am on the west coast, it's already 11:00 am on the east coast (a great time for Tom to reach people on the phone before their lunch hour). With this short list of important calls and his blue-tooth head set in his ear, Tom dials away and spends his commuting hour making 3 or 4 important calls before he even gets to his office. Now if you take this simple NET concept every day and do it with exercise, there's no excuse for you not to exercise every single day! Below are just a few examples including a few updates from the chart in my last book:

CURRENT TASK	'NET' OPPORTUNITY	'NET' SOLUTION	NOTES
Return important business calls.	Hour long commute while returning phone calls & exercising your arms.	Get a hand-grip or stress ball to work out your hands & arms each day.	Even just 10 minutes on each hand is good exercise while you're driving.
Trips to the post office, bank, etc.	Most people have to do these errands!	Walk or bicycle to do these local errands.	If you don't live within a few miles of your city center & have to drive, park your car and walk between your 'local' errands.
Entering your office building every day.	You have to get to your office every day anyway!	Change your habit of taking the elevator or escalator and instead climb the stairs every time you enter or exit the building.	Even just 2 to 3 flights of stairs is exercise you're not getting now. If your office is on a higher floor (ex: 15th floor) walk the first 5 floors & take the elevator from floor 5 up to 15. Build up endurance over time.
Going to the grocery store	Walking in and out of the store.	Instead of fighting to find a close parking spot, park at the rear of the parking lot. A brisk 1-minute walk in & out will give you an energy boost. If you don't need a	In addition to getting a quick boost of energy, you'll avoid the frustration of circling the parking lot 2 to 3 times, save time, and eliminate scratches &

		shopping cart, carry your few bags out with you.	door dings on your car!
Reading a lengthy business report.	Use this hour or two that you have to read & get exercise at the same time.	Hop on a stationary bike and get a nice workout the same time you're reading!	Most gyms have stationary bikes. There are also affordable home models as well starting at just $100.
Lunch hour.	Instead of sitting down (after sitting in your cubicle for 4 hours), walk during your lunch hour!	Get outside & walk while eating a snack or take your phone & catch up on personal calls. Grab a co-worker & make it even more fun!	You can also practice deep diaphramic breathing while walking to oxygenate your body. Your co-workers will wonder why you're so energized!
Personal phone calls to return at home.	Instead of just sitting down to return phone calls after work, utilize NET time to make it fun & get exercise!	Take your phone out to your Jacuzzi. The warm water & jets will give you a massage. If you don't have a Jacuzzi, run a hot bath & work our your upper or lower body exercise bands while making calls.	After your phone calls are made, take 15 minutes to relax &unwind. Make this your 'personal' NET time!
Read a lengthy book (for business or pleasure).	Get the book 'on tape' or download or stream an MP3.	Instead of sitting motionless while you 'read', enjoy your books while you're walking or exercising.	You'll usually retain more of your book while stimulating your physiology vs. reading in a passive state.
Brainstorm solutions to a problem.	Any time you face a problem!	Go outside for a walk while looking for solutions to your problem.	In addition to changing your venue (not sitting in your office), some fresh air &

			moving your body will help you find a solution more quickly.
Exercise & get Inspired.	While going for a run.	If you're going for a run or bike ride just for exercise, spend 10 to 15 minutes shouting out Incantations!	By repeating incantations over and over while doing physical exercise, you'll get inspired!
Watching your favorite TV show.	Instead of just being a couch potato, get your body moving!	You can ride a stationary bike while watching your favorite TV show, or do exercises & stretches during the commercials.	BONUS: in addition to getting NET exercise, you'll most likely stop the bad practice of snacking while sitting on the couch!
Planning your day, week, etc.	Get out of your office and start walking!	By walking outdoors, you'll often come up with fresh new ideas to plan tasks for the upcoming day or week while exercising.	Instead of writing your 'To Do' list on pen & paper, dictate notes to a digital recorder or your Siri while they're fresh. Finalize these notes when you're back at your office.

The very latest trend in body movement are the new 'treadmill desks'. Instead of providing an expensive office chair for their employees to sit down for eight hours each day, Salo (a financial trading company in Minnesota) has implemented a test with treadmills, which butt right up to their employee's desks where they can use their computer and talk on the phone. The employees plod along at a very slow pace (normally just 1 or 2 mph), and initial feedback is that the employees have great energy all day long, are more alert, and one employee even lost 25 lbs. in the first few months! Talk about the epitome of NET time... these folks are getting great exercise all day long while doing their work. As mentioned in a previous chapter, I built my own raised desk at my home office, so often I'll be standing while working which burns more calories, boosts my energy, and raises my productivity - the perfect health trifecta! Even when I'm super busy (last month I was on the road 20 days with speaking engagements and book signing events), I always have my precious hours at home carefully mapped out. Instead of walking around the neighborhood to do all my important errands (bank, post office, UPS store, Office Depot, grocery store), I'll hop on my bike and handle all these errands just as quickly as if I were to drive, but will get a good hour of exercise in at the same time. In Denmark (one of the healthiest countries in the world), the Danish Government has common sense policies to encourage all their citizens to ride bikes. In Copenhagen, over 40% of the city's population rides bikes! That's almost half of all their citizens riding bikes to work, to do errands, to deliver packages, or just for fun. It's no coincidence that the last time I was in Copenhagen for a diabetes conference, I did not see a single overweight person! I know it's hard to believe, but since the majority of Denmark's citizens eat much healthier and the majority of the citizens of Copenhagen exercise every single day, it actually makes sense. Many U.S. cities are now putting in more bike lanes and making it easier and safer for bicyclists, so there's never been a better time to start riding your bike again, or get a bike if you don't have one. If you're tight on cash, look on Craig's List or scope out a garage sale where you can find a decent, used bike for very little money. There's also a new movie out called "Bikes vs. Cars" and if you want to get inspired to start riding your bike again, check it out. Another option is getting a Mobile Trainer to come to you! I first heard about this concept when I was working in Las Vegas and I noticed a beautiful, very fit woman get out of her car with a large magnet sign that read: "Mobile Trainer - I Come to You". What a brilliant concept and a perfect solution to the many parents who both have full time jobs and then have to race home to work to feed and care for their children. I spoke to (who had the sign on her car) and asked about her business. Annette said in addition to working with couples with busy schedules, she also has several clients who home school their children. While the mother(s) is (are) giving assignments or tests, Annette is right in the kitchen (or the living room) training the mom and sometimes even the kids after their lessons! Annette also has a few elderly clients who don't have the will power or the energy to drive to the gym multiple times each week. Annette found that before her clients started training with her, they almost always had the same two excuses: 1) Either they claimed they "didn't have the time" to work out or 2) They were simply "too exhausted" after a long day of work. With Annette coming right to her client's house (or business) and working around their busy schedules, it works out great. In addition to saving the commute time to and from a busy gym, her clients get motivation and expert advice from a certified personal trainer. If you live in the Las Vegas area, check her service out at www.annettesfitnessfirst.com or do a Google search for a mobile trainer in your area. There's probably someone in your area who can work with you and your busy schedule at an affordable price. This makes a lot of sense especially when we're talking about your precious time and your own health. After all, what kind of price can you put on your health and/or your valuable time? These are just a few examples of how you can easily get exercise while doing other tasks in 'No Extra Time'. This principle will change your life and get your body moving in the direction of better health. If you ever find yourself thinking: "I just don't have the time to exercise", don't ever let yourself make that excuse! Implement this powerful daily strategy and I promise it will change your life forever!

ACTION ITEM 28.0

List your Top 10 items you need 'To Do' today. This could include going to the grocery store or the post office, making important phone calls, going to your office, reading a report, helping a friend do some errands, etc. Pick ONE item you need to do and combine some form of exercise while you're doing that task. The easiest tip I give my clients on their first day is when they go to work. Park at the far end of the parking lot and do a brisk walk into the office and then when they get there, bypass the elevator and walk up the stairs to their office floor. This usually won't take any more time (perhaps an extra 1 to 2 minutes), but will provide you some quick exercise (and a boost of energy) in 'No Extra Time'. If you work at home, pick at least one important phone call you have on your list and make that phone call while walking around the block.

Tomorrow, you can map out a few extra items you can also do using this important new principle!

Chapter 29.
The Best and Easiest Exercise? Walking!

While swimming is considered one of the best and most ideal exercises because of the low impact on your joints, I feel walking is the best and easiest exercise, since not everyone has access to a swimming pool. Anybody and everybody has access to the ground. Most everybody can walk even if you're 100 years old and using a cane or a walker, you can still shuffle down a sidewalk or hallway somewhere. If you're not fortunate to still have your legs, you can still roll your wheelchair to get exercise. The important point is to *move* every single day. I've heard all the excuses why people can't walk (or exercise): "I live in a cold climate", "I don't live near any parks", "It's dark outside before I leave and after I get home from work", "I don't live in a safe neighborhood where I can walk". I've literally heard every excuse in the book. I believe there's always an opportunity to walk and that's why walking is the best exercise because it's the one exercise you can easily do every single day. Now let's look at some of these excuses like living in an extreme cold climate like Alaska in the winter - you can warm up and stretch inside the house for a few minutes and put on multiple layers and even a face mask if it's below 0°. If it's raining, put on a raincoat or use an umbrella and walk to the store. If you get a few raindrops on you, remember your body is comprised of 75% water, so a few drops won't melt you. If you don't have access to a park or a safe neighborhood to walk, you can often find a shopping mall or a large building to walk inside the hallways. In some malls (like the Mall of America in Minneapolis), there are avid walking groups that take advantage of being indoors during their snowy, cold winter months. For people who use the excuse of it being too dark in the morning before work, that excuse is now invalid with the invention of great products like the Night Runner 270° lights which clip onto your running sneakers or walking shoes to light your way and keep you safe. If you want to stay healthy, you can figure out how to walk every day. After reading the preceding NET exercise chapter, there's no excuse not to walk every day. You can always find some activity that you have to do every day anyway like making a phone call, going to the post office or bank, shopping at the grocery store, etc. If you're traveling and stuck sitting on different airplanes for most of the day, you can do airplane aerobics in your seat including miniature steps with your feet in place. Unlike most airline passengers I see who get off one flight and plop right back down at a seat near their gate, I make it a priority on airport layovers to walk around the entire airport at a brisk pace. I do this while I'm returning the phone calls I've received during the flight. Even just 15 to 20 minutes of walking gives me you a nice boost of energy. Another tip is to surround yourself with friends or family members who are open-minded to exercise, or at least to walking. One of the most common questions you'll hear in my family's household is: "Do you want to go for a walk?" This could be in the morning while we're planning the day's family activities, or it could be after lunch to help burn off a few calories. One of the other great things about walking and why it's the perfect exercise is that you can even walk alone. It's not necessarily a team sport or activity. I remember years ago reading a physiology book, which described several different animal species and how they adapted over the years to move their bodies. Snakes of course contract their body and use thousands of scales to slither on the ground and climb trees. Horses have incredibly powerful legs to gallop at speeds of over 40 mph. Ducks not only have wings to fly, but they have wide webbed feet to effortlessly propel themselves on the surface of the water. If you look at the earliest Homo sapiens (and our earlier predecessors Homo erectus), our flat feet with five toes were designed to hold us upright and walk very easily and naturally. Walking is what our bodies were designed to do. Our bodies were never created or designed to sit motionless in our cars for an hour commute to an office to then sit motionless for eight hours and then come home to sit motionless on a couch for three hours before lying down flat in our beds for another 6 to 8 hours. It is vitally important that you make walking not only a priority, but that you figure out a way to walk at least 15 to 30 minutes a day. Once you incorporate walking into your daily lifestyle you'll start reaping some of the many benefits including a dozen right here:

1) Burning excess calories to help maintain a healthy weight.

2) Preventing or helping prevent heart disease, high blood pressure and many other diseases.

3) Improving your circulation.

4) Stimulating your lymphatic system and boosting your immune system.

5) Strengthening your bones, muscles, joints and tendons.

6) Increasing your energy.

7) Instantly improving or enhancing your mood.

8) Improving your sleep and sleep patterns.

9) Improving your balance and coordination.

10) Increasing your mental alertness.

11) Lowering the risk and effects of Alzheimer's, and

12) Simply making you feel better!

The most important benefit and the key reason to walk every day is the proven fact by every single study that walking leads to a longer life. Research at the University of Michigan Medical School reports "Those who exercise regularly in their 50's and 60's who have underlying health conditions are 45% less likely to die over the next eight years than their non-walking counterparts"! [29-1] According to The Independent, a daily walk can add seven years to your life! [29-2]

ACTION ITEM 29.0

Set a goal that you're going to start walking every single day. Start walking TODAY while you're returning a short phone call. Once you start this habit and increase the time you walk every day, it will become a daily addiction as you start to feel better and enjoy increased energy!

SECTION III: Your Outlook and Faith

"Happiness is an attitude.
We either make ourselves miserable, or
happy and strong. The amount
of work is the same."
- Francesca Reigler

Chapter 30.
What are Your Priorities?

Sometimes in my health seminars, I ask audience members what areas of their lives are most important to them? I'll cue the audience by throwing out a few suggestions including family-life (or marriage), career, friendships, finances, contribution, God, etc. and eventually someone will yell out 'health'! That gets a good laugh from the audience since everyone in the room is attending a 'Health' seminar. It's easy to get caught up with work obligations, errands, paying bills, and other 'to do's' that we often forget to focus on our own health. Ask any person on their deathbed if they have any regrets? If you talk with them long enough, the most common thing dying people wish they had was their health. Sometimes, they will pray for a few more months, or a few more years of their life to spend with family members or close friends. You never hear about anyone reflecting during their last living days or wishing they had "made more money", "worked harder at the office", or "gained more material possessions". Take another example: if you've ever been in a bad car accident or gone through a major operation where you couldn't get out of bed for a week or longer, or if you've ever had a debilitating back or neck injury, my guess is you would trade *anything* to regain your health. When your perfect health is jeopardized or taken away from you (even for a short period of time), that's usually when we most appreciate it. Yet most people (in the U.S. anyway) take health for granted. Don't believe me? Why is 2/3rds of the U.S. population now obese? Why do we have far more people on prescription drugs and painkillers than any other country in the world? I don't think anyone consciously neglects or ignores their health on purpose. Many people are working longer hours for less money, have more demands on their time, and are under more stress. Combine that added pressure with lengthy commutes to and from the office and the excuse for not focusing on our health is always the same: "I don't have the time to exercise". With people tethered to their computers, smart phones and smart watches, there seems to be less private time and more non-stop demands from e-mails, tweets, texts, IM's, PM's, social media requests, let alone phone calls! Here's a news flash...unless you prioritize time <u>every day</u> for yourself and your health, things will never change. One of the reasons I started waking up at 4:30 am is that I often start my workday very early and couldn't always find the time to exercise. When I'm acting, I sometimes have to be on set by 6:00 am, which means I have to leave for work by 5:15 am or 5:30 am. I used to find myself making the same excuse: "I just don't have the time to exercise", especially getting home 15 or 16 hours after I left. One of the reasons the studios and networks pay actors a lot of money is that actors often work very long days (12 to 16 hours), and when shooting a film an actor may be away from home for months at a time. The daily work on a film set is not as glamorous as it looks in the finished movie when you're working those long hours. An important (life-changing) decision I made several years ago was that I'd exercise <u>every single morning</u> no matter what. I did not allow myself any more excuses! The ideal amount of time to get a good work out in (to really energize your body and jump start your metabolism) is 30 minutes and that's what I strive for every morning. But for those days when I have a very early call time, or a super early flight to attend a book signing event or seminar, I still squeeze in at least 15 to 20 minutes of exercise in no matter what. Often times it may be just 15 minutes of push ups, sit ups, crunches, leg lifts, etc. Other times it might be 20 minutes of jumping jacks combined with some jump rope, but for the past seven years, I've exercised first thing every single morning. On the very rare occasion when I don't work out first thing in the morning (usually when traveling on a cross country red-eye flight), I feel sluggish, lethargic and simply not as mentally sharp as when I exercise first thing to do very morning. The best way to prioritize your health is to make excellent health your # 1 Goal. Tony Robbins says: "Make whatever you really want (in this case your good health) a 'Must' instead of just a 'Should'." In my research for this book (which has included meeting with over 16,500 individuals one-on-one about their health), the rare 3 to 5% who take no prescription drugs, appear to be very fit, have excellent skin and a noticeable positive energy about them. They all prioritize their health in some way. It could be something as simple as making sure they go for a walk every day, or perhaps a commitment to have a salad or a serving of green vegetables at every meal. As mentioned earlier in this book, these like-minded people are not health fanatics, but they all prioritize some sort of exercise (even just walking or biking) at least five days a week as well as watching what foods they consume (at least 80% of the time). They make this a priority! I could make a list of hundreds of people I've worked with who have radically turned their health around in just 7 to 10 days. When I say radical, I mean a 10 to 20 lb. weight loss, noticeably clearer skin, improved allergies, lower blood pressure, lower cholesterol, etc. Not only Ronald Farnham, but Bruce Ellington, Andrew Reilly, Desmond Bailey, Vanessa Esperanza, Peter Allport, Rob Baker, Phil and Willie Jones, but hundreds of others. Of these 500+ people, many of them actually knew what to do in terms of diet, exercise, etc. but not all of them decided to make health an absolute 'priority'. The reason I picked 7 days for our "Alkalize & Energize" cleanse (instead of 30 or 60 days) is that most people are willing to prioritize their health for that short amount of time. If people can get really impressive results (which they all do) within a week, they're usually excited to continue for another few days, weeks, or months with health as their 'priority'. The end goal is to make health a *lifelong priority*. It has worked for me as I'm hooked for life on feeling excellent every day! I love what TV talk show host Elisabeth Hasselbeck once said: "Nobody's life is ever all balanced. It's a conscious decision to choose your priorities every day."

Another reason to prioritize your health is that with great health comes more energy and stamina to ultimately help achieve all of your secondary priorities and goals. Going back to the big easel pad exercise I do in some of my health seminars, I put a challenge out to the audience to find *any* priority that does not benefit from you having optimum health and energy? Nobody has found one yet. You can't give 100% to your career if you're tired and in poor health. You can't give as much love and attention to your wife and kids if you're fighting the flu or feeling run down. Most people won't spend extra time on their personal dreams and ambitions if they've run out of energy at the end of the day. Decide right now that you're going to prioritize your health no matter how small the step or action you take. Perhaps the first step is to announce to your

family that you're going to give up your nightly ice cream ritual and slowly change or replace your other bad diet habits. The fact of telling your family is leverage and if they're supportive they'll want to see you succeed and help hold you accountable. If you live alone, tell your co-workers or a good friend about your health goals. Better yet, get a coach to help you achieve your priorities and reach your goals. Whatever priorities you choose, I wish you the very best of luck and hope it's your first small step towards reclaiming the perfect health you deserve!

ACTION ITEM 30.0

List out your Top 3 priorities in your life. If Health is not one of them, decide today that health will be one of your Top priorities (if not your # 1 priority). Write down in your journal or on your smart phone what step(s) you'll start taking today towards excellent health! Perhaps you start using a website or an app. like www.myfitnesspal.com. Or maybe you decide for the next 7 days you're going to walk for 15 minutes every morning and make it a priority!

Chapter 31.
The Mind-Body Connection

At University of Minnesota's Center for Spirituality and Healing, Mind-Body specialist Dr. James Gordon states: "The mind and body are essentially inseparable: the brain and peripheral nervous system, the endocrine and immune systems, and indeed, all the organs of our body and all the emotional responses we have, share a common chemical language and are constantly communicating with one another". In plain English, what goes on in your mind has a direct effect or impact on the rest of your body. Most people have heard of a placebo effect. To clarify for those who may not fully understand the term, a placebo is a fairly common simulated or otherwise medically ineffectual treatment (like a sugar pill) for a disease or other medical condition intended to deceive the patient. A person given such an ineffectual treatment (the sugar pill) will often have a perceived or actual improvement in their condition commonly called the placebo effect or placebo response. Placebos can produce some objective physiological changes, such as changes in heart rate, blood pressure, energy and enhanced chemical activity in the brain. The 'nocebo' effect is a newer scientific term used to describe the phenomenon in which inert substances or mere suggestions of substances bring about negative (adverse) effects in a patient. Ty Bollinger and several doctors in his documentary film series "The Truth About Cancer" discuss a common example, which happens often today in oncology offices. To hear the three words "You have cancer" must be horrific enough, but an example of a nocebo effect is when an oncologist tells a patient their cancer is metastatic or stage IV cancer, and that they may only have six more months to live. The nocebo effect from the patient's mind to their body (and their state of health) can change dramatically and fast! Before heading to the local pharmacy, you should be aware there are many natural alternatives (actual natural hormones and chemicals) your body can manufacture and deliver for free! Dr. Deepak Chopra who taught at the medical schools of Tufts University, Boston University and Harvard University and later became Chief of Staff at the New England

Memorial Hospital before establishing a private practice, talks often about the mind-body connection. In his books the consistent message Dr. Chopra delivers and the advice he gives to patients is to understand through meditation, focus, and positive thoughts, your endocrine glands can often produce for free "the equivalent prescriptions in your own body's internal pharmacy vs. purchasing synthetic prescription drugs from the retail pharmacy". Your internal, natural hormones such as adrenaline, cortisol and others can be just as effective as an expensive prescription purchased at your local Walgreen's pharmacy, for $0. A great example is the hormone oxytocin that acts primarily as a neuromodulator in the brain and is best known its roles in sexual reproduction in females, in particular during and after childbirth. It's released in large amounts after distension of the cervix and uterus during labor, facilitating birth. Unlocking your internal pharmacy starts with positive emotions including but not limited to: love (by the far the most powerful), humor, optimism, and hope. Triggers can also include: nature, pets, playing, music, movies, poetry, and hobbies that you are passionate or excited about.[31-1] If you'd like to give meditation a try, there are now several great websites (and apps) where you can access hundreds of hours of guided and unguided exercises that will do wonders for the well being of your entire body. Think of it like a gym membership for your mind. Some of these apps are free and others offer free trials and if you like any of them, you can continue for just a few dollars a month. The best apps I've found in my research include: www.Calm.com, www.Mindful.org, www.Headspace.com to name a few. That's a small price to pay for peace of mind!

Also, don't forget to laugh! There are thousands of case studies that have been done with laughter especially in patients by Dr. Norman Cousins, who has been called the father of laughter therapy medicine. Dr. Cousins treated his own pain from many ailments including his life-threatening joint disease with a 10-minute daily dose of laughter. Laughter decreases stress hormones and increases immune cells and infection-fighting antibodies, thus improving your body's resistance to disease. Laughter also triggers the release of endorphins, the body's natural feel-good chemicals. If after a really long laughing spell, you feel really good, energized and even relieved of possible body pain or negative thoughts, that is because of the naturally created and released endorphins in your body. There are even laughter groups, clubs, and associations all around the country where people get together to laugh and feel good! Another excellent example of the mind-body connection is demonstrated by Jack Canfield (famous author of the Chicken Soup for the Soul books). At many of Jack's live seminars and events, he'll ask for a volunteer from the audience to come up on stage. Jack then asks the volunteer to hold his or her arms straight out to their side. Jack tells this audience member to repeat out loud several empowering phrases and then from behind Jack will push his weight down on this individual's arms to try and force the arms down usually to no avail. Jack waits a moment, has the same person shake his or her arms out and asks them to clear their head. Jack once again tells this audience member to repeat some phrases (this time negative or disempowering). Once again Jack pushes all his weight down on this individual's arms and this time both the audience member's arms go down quite easily! Most medical doctors believe in the power of medicines and surgery as the first course of action, but recently more doctors and even some surgeons are becoming open minded to the plethora of options to let the body heal itself, which under ideal circumstances (with an excellent diet, enough exercise, and proper rest) can work wonders. It's common sense that if all the other animals in the world can heal themselves without synthetic prescription drugs, you should be able to heal yourself as well with your own internal drugs that your body manufactures for free. Just remember that almost everything manufactured in your body (good and bad) usually starts in the mind! Here's some food for thought I'll end this chapter on: Have you ever noticed if you're focused on negative thoughts and get into a really angry state, that it can take quite a while (sometimes hours) to get back to a happy, grateful or energetic state? Tony Robbins, who has been studying the mind-body connection for decades, explains: "If you are angry for just 5 minutes, your biochemistry radically changes and it can take up to 4 to 5 hours to change your body chemistry back!" [31-2] Wow...that's a pretty powerful incentive to shift your mindset (what you focus on) to carefully consider the people in your daily life, and watch for any outside stimuli that might put you in a negative, angry state. There's nothing wrong with getting angry or upset once in a while for a short time - it happens to all of us. Just don't stay in that stressed out, angry state for more than a minute or two as what happens in your mind directly affects your body for longer than we realize!

ACTION ITEM 31.0
Do your *own* research to find another example of a powerful mind-body connection exercise that you can try, or perhaps download one of the mediation apps above to start meditating today!

Chapter 32.
Your Beliefs, Thoughts and Perceptions

Belief - be·lief (bə'lēf) noun: belief; plural noun: beliefs 1. An acceptance that a statement is true or that something exists. Ex. "his belief in the value of hard work".

With the definition of Belief explained above, let me share with you a few of the disturbing comments I heard at health benefit fairs the past two years. Most of these people were retirees ranging in age from their 50's to 70's. I cringed inside when these people told me their 'beliefs' with such certainty. These powerful beliefs will affect many of these people for the rest of their lives! However, my job was strictly to help answer questions about their prescription drugs. I'm just sharing exactly what I heard...

- A 62-year-old lady came to the Express Scripts table concerned about her husband who just got diagnosed with early onset diabetes. The doctor told them he "Would have to take his new medication for the rest of his life."

- A 55-year-old HR person (hosting a benefits fair in Southern California) had breast cancer, a heart attack, and was now taking 10 prescriptions each day. She claimed: "I've been cursed with bad genes!"

- A lady came to my table remarking that her husband's cardiologist said unequivocally: "He would be on Crestor and Plavix for the rest of his life."

- A lady (in her mid 50's) taking several prescriptions confided to me: "I just hope I live until I'm 70."

- A 60-year-old lady (close to retirement and on no prescriptions yet) remarked: "I'll probably need to be taking some prescriptions very soon."

- A 62-year-old gentleman bragged: "Oh my wife is <u>very</u> healthy. She only takes two daily prescriptions."

- A 57-year-old retiree told me: "My wife died of cancer. We all knew she was going to die early due to her bad genes. Not one of her female family members ever lived past 52."

- A newly retired gentleman remarked: "Since I just turned 65, my doctor had to put me on cholesterol medication like he recommends for all his retired patients."

- A gentleman (in his 50's) walked up to my table complaining about the high costs of his drugs: "My doctor said I cannot take any generic prescriptions."

- A nurse (and a patient aide) who unpacks all of a new patient's things when they're admitted to the Northern California hospital where I was attending a benefits fair, commented: "I sometimes sort through 20 or more prescriptions that patients bring in".

- A 35-year-old man told me: "I'm too young to take prescriptions now, but I'll definitely need to start taking them in about 10 years."

In order to accept that any statement is true, we draw from our references and/or past experiences over a period of time. The 'belief' that most people today have about prescription drugs (and how 'normal' it has become for people to be taking daily prescriptions) comes from the media, hundreds of thousands of commercials, print and online advertisements, billboards, etc. that we are constantly exposed to. This is true for current prescription drugs and for the thousands of 'over the counter' drugs, which required a prescription just a few years ago. It's really disturbing to see that young kids are now popping pills like candy! If you don't believe me, just go to any public middle or high school and ask any teacher how many of their students are on prescription drugs? (ADD, ADHD meds, anti-depressants, anti-anxiety pills, diabetes meds, pain medications, asthma medications, allergy prescriptions, etc.) My point is that the belief (perception) about prescription drugs is much different than it was for people growing up 50 years ago and today's kids are practically programmed to think that taking a few prescription drugs each day is totally normal! This new prescription drug culture gets reinforced at work, within the household, etc. to the point where it's practically expected to take a least a few prescription drugs every day in the U.S. and more and more pills as you get older. The common perception (which I've experienced while speaking at hundreds of health benefit fairs) is that "it's just part of the natural aging process, where our old, frail bodies need a few more pills to work better". Let me get back to the "Super Healthy 4%" of the 16,000+ individuals I met with at my table at the health fairs on behalf of Medco and Express Scripts. These super healthy people (who looked 10 to 15 younger than their age, did not appear to be overweight, and were not taking *any* prescription drugs) had much different beliefs from the majority of the other 96%, especially when it came to the retiree groups (in their 50's, 60's, or 70's). This super-healthy, elite group was very active (walking, hiking, running... a few were even doing triathlons in their 60's and 70's) and did not see themselves as 'old'. If anything, they would admit that they were 'middle-aged', but did not put any label on themselves as being 'old' or "only having a few good years left" as I heard several other of their peers tell me. I believe that you are as old as you want to be. As soon as you start labeling yourself or letting the number of birthday candles on your cake dictate how you should act, you're in trouble. Thank God the 120-year-old man I read about yesterday in USA Today (celebrating his 12th decade doing his daily yoga) doesn't worry about that either. One tip that will greatly help you feel and act younger and healthier is to spend some of your time with *younger* friends. My oldest sister (in her 60's) has the energy, vitality and productivity of someone in her 40's and one of the reasons is she has a *lot* of younger friends (10 to 20 years younger than she is). It doesn't matter what your age is, if you're 90 and reading this book, I'm not suggesting that you dismiss all of your 90+ year old good friends (who are still alive), but honestly if that is your entire peer group, then there's a good chance you will hear other old people comment about losing another friend when they read the obituaries, complain about the high prices of their prescription drugs, moan about their aches and pains or comment about their failing memories and diminishing eyesight, etc. If you're 90 or older and you can reach out to a younger family member, friend, or neighbor or join another peer group (with people in their 60's or 70's who are active), some of that youthful activity and thinking will rub off on you. You can immediately feel the different energy level and vibe. It's almost like when the grandson comes back from summer vacation he spent with the older grandparents and the first night home at the dinner table, the father comments: "Son, you've been hanging around and listening to your damn grandfather too much!". I think you understand, but if not, Tony Robbins sums it up best with one of my favorite quotes in the world: "Your life is a direct reflection of the expectation of your peer group." That statement is *very* true. Let me share with you a 'disempowering belief'. I changed in my life a few years ago and I'm sure you see this problem every day which puts so many people in a state of overwhelm and/or stress. Of course too much stress can create havoc with one's health. There is this totally false belief that our iPads and new smart phones (with all the latest and greatest apps) are making our lives easier and connecting all of us together. Nothing could be farther from the truth! I love and embrace all the modern technologies and tools we have at our fingertips for instant communication, but they can also be the source of massive stress if not managed correctly. Let's discuss just two of the modern communication tools in particular: text messages and IM's (instant messaging). I'd estimate over 80% of the people I know keep their cell phone with them all day long and when their phone beeps, chirps or rings, they immediately check that text (or IM if linked to one of their social media accounts). They read the message and quickly reply back... at all hours, in the middle of lunch or dinner, sometimes when they're driving down the freeway! I see many problems with this type of 'constant engagement'. 1) I often see people get distracted from what they're currently working on to reply to somebody else's problem or demands, 2) I observe a lot of stress and tension people often put on themselves believing that "they must get back to this person right away", and 3) They don't allow themselves any 'downtime' to disconnect or unwind. A girl I was dating for several years was the in the import-export business and would often come by my place for dinner and/or a movie. Many times at 11:00 pm or later on a Friday night, she'd get sidetracked for 30 minutes or so with lengthy texts going back and forth. She would be totally stressed out on what was supposed to be her night off. She justified her non-stop work hours by the fact that her client was in China and they needed all the figures and information 'right now'. I could go on citing dozens of other examples of how constant text messaging has brought added stress to our lives. I admit there are unique jobs and circumstances during the workday that demand we be connected, so this strategy might not work for everybody, but here's how I manage my life and keep my sanity in this fast-paced digital world:

1) I don't check my e-mail, messages on my smart phone, or any of my social media accounts for the first two hours of my morning. That is *my* precious time to gather my thoughts, appreciate the simple things in my life I can be grateful for, focus on my goals and dreams and then outline my plan of attack for the upcoming day. As Abraham Lincoln famously said: "Give me six hours to chop down a tree and I will spend the first four sharpening the axe". When I finally do open my e-mails, start checking my text messages, IM's, social media pages in the morning (usually by 8:00 am), I'm insanely prepared and laser focused on what "I want out my day", *not* what "other people want me to respond to."

2) The other habit that I've installed over the past few years (which has made me extremely productive while helping eliminate stress), is I scan over all my messages, e-mails, etc. and instantly reply to all the ones I can handle in 1 to 2 minutes. For the more involved, detailed responses or actions required answering my different partners, clients, vendors, etc. I'll write out a priority list (ex. A,B,C) and then handle them as needed throughout the day (or possibly the next day). The most important 'belief' I live by when checking texts during the day, is that I no longer need to immediately reply to texts, unless it is truly an emergency or an urgent situation. Over 60% of the texts and IM's I receive do *not* need an immediate response from me, so I'm not going to let any of those distract me from my top priorities for the day. I had a client challenge me on this philosophy once and she was insistent that her boss and her team members expected immediate text responses from her during business hours (which for her could range from 7:00 am to 8:00 pm). In essence, she was supposed to be at someone else's beck

and call for up to 13 hours a day! I asked her a few questions about what types of messages these were and found out that most of her texts in fact were *not* urgent or emergencies that needed to be handled or responded to immediately. We discussed in detail how she could better handle this matter. I told her the next time she met with her boss, she should have a professional discussion about his beliefs and expectations about the dozens of e-mails and text messages flying back and forth all hours of the day. She approached her boss with a proposal that she would respond to *all* of his texts and IM's by the very end of the day, and would respond immediately if there was a text that was urgent to their mutual goals or business at hand. The same applies to co-workers. You could have this same discussion at your next team meeting and you might find the whole toxic, stressful, working-vibe changes for the better. I also coached her to have fun with this exercise. The next time one of her co-workers sends her a text to 'REPLY ASAP', with her brand new 'belief', she could smile and say to herself: "How dare they!" and not worry about the message until later in the day when she chose to reply. What happened the next few weeks was almost a miracle. My client's productivity went through the roof as she was no longer distracted (or side tracked) dozens of times each day and the quality of her work actually improved. She also gained back a calm and peace of mind that she hadn't experienced in years and her blood pressure (which was slightly high) dropped significantly! All by changing her beliefs and false assumptions.

Here's another example about how 'beliefs and perceptions' can affect one's health. In the Miami VA system (which serves 175,000 veterans), it was recently reported that doctors were able to significantly lower blood pressure in 100 veterans living in underserved areas by using Telemedicine appointments alone.[32-1] I found this very interesting that simply from hearing a doctor's voice and having someone listen to the patient's problems and medical needs, these doctors were able to lower blood pressure long distance! I'm a big proponent of using technology like the telephone, internet chats, and even video conferencing to allow doctors to reach out and communicate with more patients. It saves both parties a lot of time and expense, and in many cases doctors can update their patient's prescriptions, share test or lab results, or simply check in with them. The most important thing for the patient is the 'belief' that their doctors take the time to show they care! What happens when you have a strong enough belief or thought? That can often lead to one of the most important aspects determining one's health... Faith!

ACTION ITEM 32.0

If you *believe* you have to immediately respond to the daily barrage of text messages, phone calls, e-mails, or IM's every day, make an honest assessment of how many are truly urgent? Set up a meeting with your boss, co-workers, or perhaps your family members and set new rules that you'll only immediately respond to urgent messages in a timely manner. If that's not possible, then set up new guidelines where you'll no longer immediately respond to message before _____am or after _____pm. You'll find after doing this exercise that much of the stress and pressure you put on yourself was a false 'belief'.

Chapter 33.
Your Outlook and Faith

Your outlook (backed by some sort of faith) determines almost everything in your life including your health. Do you have an optimistic outlook, or are you a skeptic who sees the glass as 'half empty'? You literally need to have faith to make it through each day. Consider a few daily examples: you must have absolute faith that when you're driving to work that the other drivers coming straight at you from the opposite direction traveling 55 mph won't swerve a foot across the yellow lines and crash into you. If you're taking the subway or train, you must have faith that the tunnels below the earth (and in some cases way underneath rivers, lakes or mountains) won't cave in and crush you. When you get to your office in the morning, you must have faith that the elevator will work properly and that the cable suspending your elevator car doesn't break. These days if you go out to any public place, you must have faith that a radical terrorist won't start shooting at you. Those of you with lofty goals and ambitions also need to have faith. When you set high goals (out of your comfort zone), at first you don't know exactly how you're going to achieve some of your biggest goals or highest dreams. But you have faith that over the course of time, you'll overcome obstacles, learn new skills, and somehow stretch your limits to achieve your goals! No matter what your background, education, income level, or past experiences, life is not always easy. This includes many health challenges along with aging that *will* occur. Having different 'beliefs' (as mentioned in the previous chapter) is important, as is your daily outlook or faith.

I recently had the opportunity to interview **Nicole Abisinio** who is the founder of Gabriel's Messenger Ministries and a spiritual coach and speaker. In addition to coaching people to help them find their faith, Nicole has certain rituals she practices every day herself. First thing every morning when she wakes up, she thanks God and prays. Nicole stays very quiet and asks God to help her be a better person, shine his light, and help her make a difference in other people's lives. This quiet time in the morning includes no television or radio in order to eliminate possible negative programming. At her Ministry, Nicole hosts a live event called 'Pure Power' with topics including: Restocking the Kitchen (renewing your mind), Strength Training (forgiveness), Stamina Building (7 ways to pray powerfully) and Sculpting (fasting). Nicole who is also a successful film producer and actress recently transitioned into her current role after doing some soul-searching. Ten years prior, Nicole was very busy working as an actor and model and *thought* she was healthy. In fact, she was eating healthy, worked out six days a week, and looked healthy, but it was all superficial because she wasn't healthy on the inside. She faced constant pressures from casting directors, producers, and her peers about her looks, figure, and wardrobe. Nicole was so busy working on her *outside* and chasing after man-made material items and recognition that she neglected her *inside* spirit. Like many of us, Nicole used to hold on to anger, resentment, and had not yet learned how to be truly forgiving. How we handle these negative emotions can have a huge impact on our emotional, mental and physical health. She occasionally went to church and believed in God, but didn't understand and fully connect with the Lord until she read The Bible. That's where she found God and internal peace. Nicole found her faith, which included forgiveness. All the inner turmoil she held onto inside was not healthy. Today Nicole is a healthy, complete person on the inside and outside. During the time in Nicole's life when she was very busy acting and modeling, she did not enjoy the incredible health and peace of mind that she enjoys today. It was when she found her faith and her inner peace that changed her life. Nicole hasn't had to go to a doctor for any illness in eight years, whereas before she was often at the doctor's office being treated for illnesses and ailments. She admits to having gotten the flu a handful of times, but she literally "prayed and it left me in Jesus's name". She consistently prays (coming from a place of gratitude) and to this day has lived a healthy life. The spiritual healing is the reason why she doesn't need to see doctors for being ill or sickness anymore with the exception of an occasional preventative check-up. In fact her most recent blood test results came back as perfect! A few tips Nicole offers everybody:

1) You have to be careful what you feed your mind.

2) Surround yourself with positive people.

3) Get out of yourself by helping others, and

4) Realize that you have the ability to make things better if you have faith in God.

Nicole sums up the importance of a positive outlook by stating: "The sickness in the body is often a reflection of the sickness in the mind, heart, and soul. Focusing on being a blessing to others on a daily basis helps the mind, heart and soul to be productive, selfless and healthy."

One of the most incredible stories of faith and healing (there are many out there) is the story of my good friend **Tony Davis**. There have been numerous television specials about Tony's incredible story. In a world filled with violence and hatred, Tony Davis stood out as a man who gave to those in need. Through an ironic twist of fate, Tony unknowingly became a target in an ongoing gang war while out one night in Los Angeles and was shot multiple times and left for dead! Tony's life would never be the same. He miraculously survived and spent several weeks in the hospital. With his voice gone and a leg in need of amputation, Tony turned to God. What came after (and documented by the paramedics, his doctors and hospital staff) is known as "The Miracle of Tony Davis" of which I was honored to be a producer for the documentary film about his life.

While Nicole and Tony are Christians, the similar message of faith applies to all religions including the Jewish faith and even Buddhism. Buddhism came from the teachings of the wise Siddhartha Gautama who believed life is permeated with suffering caused by desire and that suffering ceases when desire ceases. Furthermore that enlightenment can come when one can be liberated from it by mental and moral self-purification. In essence, look *inward* and not outward at all of the modern world desires, trappings and material objects which don't guarantee happiness. Meditation and having a quiet time each day are a big part of this religion. So what if you're not a religious person and you never go to church, temple,

mosque, etc.? To find inner peace and to help find a balance of health, I think it's healthy to believe in some force greater than yourself and certainly larger than man. Perhaps you believe in the 'Universe'; some higher level to be respected, to have appreciation of faith and to be grateful for? Having a positive outlook and faith is the key to a happy, successful life. For anyone with a serious life threatening illness, cancer, etc., faith can be a matter of life and death! Take the severe and most awful news nobody ever wants to hear from a doctor: "You have terminal cancer and you only have six months to live." It's fascinating to me that certain people will take those words to heart and become a victim of the cancer diagnosis, while other people will reach deep into their soul to awaken something within them and will not accept the diagnosis, or certainly not accept the short time-line of life they've been prescribed. These people (and you may know some friends or family members who beat cancer or greatly extended their time) defy the expectations of the medical community by unwavering faith. Having faith and saying prayers for people's health is such powerful medicine that many hospitals have some sort of chapel where patients and/or their loved ones can pray. In conclusion, having a negative outlook and worrying all the time creates stress, which can lead to illness. That stress (which often creates acid) can cause havoc on your body and perpetuate a state of illness and despair, as we know from the powerful mind-body connection. One of the biggest lessons I learned that changed my life (in addition to trying to always have a positive outlook and faith) is not worry about anything beyond my control. I can't change the weather *outside*, but I can control the weather *inside,* which is my positive outlook and faith every day!

ACTION ITEM 33.0
Identify one item that happens today which is 'beyond your control'. An example would be a reckless, rude driver who cuts you off. Identify that you cannot control what other people may do. Pray for them and go on with your day, not allowing someone or something else to influence your

positive outlook on your upcoming happy and productive day!

Chapter 34.
The 'Boob Tube' Trap

First of all, it would be hypocritical of me to preach to anyone *not* to watch television, as that's the business I work in. My mom years ago used to call the television set the 'boob tube' referencing the stupid, lethargic state people often end up in after sitting motionless and staring at the television set for hours at a time. The looming problem in our current society is that the average American now watches five hours of TV per day! [34-1] Many children watch more than six or seven hours each day! Five hours per day works out to 35 hours per week. That's almost a 40 hour work week sitting sedentary and getting programmed by someone else's messages! It should be obvious that sitting on a couch or a Lazy-Boy recliner virtually motionless for hours at a time is not healthy. There are now multiple studies that conclude sitting too long actually shortens your life span, as mentioned in a previous chapter. The double whammy is that often times, people watching TV late at night will make their television watching a 'special event' complete with a big bowl of popcorn, some soda, perhaps a large bowl of ice cream while others might guzzle a few beers. It's common sense that the act of sitting still while consuming large amounts of calories late at night before you retire to bed (also motionless) is not the smartest way to stay fit, trim and energetic.

The other problem with watching too much television is the way it affects people's minds and emotional states. People who feed their mind with positive, educational books or listen to inspirational audio programs of their favorite success coaches can change their emotional state including their biochemistry. Others who meditate with specially selected background music are choosing to program their minds in a different way that also changes their emotional state in a positive way while improving their overall physical state. When you sit down in front of the 'boob tube', you're often being programmed with information that's often negative or depressing. A great example of this is the majority of Americans who wake up every morning and first thing they do is turn on their television sets. Every morning, millions of Americans get bombarded with news on the television, and later on the radio for those who commute to work. It's understandable to see how many people have a negative point of view of how terrible things are in the world when they've been *programmed* with an abundance of negative news for 30 to 60 minutes each morning. Even the tone of the Weather Channel (which many people watch in the morning as they start their day) has changed over the years. It doesn't just broadcast the standard weather report anymore, but often promotes gripping headlines such as: "Worst Flooding in 50 Years Could Kill Thousands!", "Looming California Earthquake Could Wipe Out Entire Cities.", or "Fiery Inferno Could Change the State's Landscape as We Know it!" I think you get the picture and I'm not faulting the news stations or the Weather Channel for sensationalizing their programs as every channel has to compete to get viewers these days. I'm not suggesting you never watch or listen to the news or the weather, but if you program your mind each morning with negative, depressing, and sometimes politically distorted news, this is not healthy for your emotional state. By focusing your attention on natural disasters, wars, terrorism, unemployment, the banking crisis, our failing schools, rising unemployment, local murders in your town, another huge oil spill, spiking gas prices, political scandals, bank robberies, the current health epidemic, the national debt of our country as well as other floundering economies around the world, etc., this is an insane way to start your day with the right mindset! Here are a few statistics to ponder: The January 2007 publication "Lawyers and Settlements" reported that the U.S. market for antidepressants accounted for 66% of the entire global market vs. 23% in Europe and 11% for the rest of the world.[34-2] 66% of consumption of the world's antidepressant medication by a single country is insane! We could learn a lesson from the Fijians who are considered by many to be the happiest people in the world. Fiji is far from the richest country in the world, but the Fijian people are doing many of tips mentioned in this book and are consistently happy. Here's another jaw dropping statistic: from 1988 to 2008, the rate of antidepressant use in the U.S. among all ages increased nearly 400%! [34-3] This included the exponential growth market in teenage antidepressants with the study including those children and teens 12 to 17 years old. In 1985 sales of antidepressants in the U.S. were just $240 million and in 2004 sales were an astounding $11.2 billion, with some people estimating that the revenues for antidepressants in the US could surpass $15 billion in a few years! Common sense should dictate that taking pills is not always the answer. So what is the answer? Try cutting back the hours of television you watch every day, perhaps from 5 hours to 2 hours (to start with). Be cognizant of what programs you're watching and ask yourself: "Is there a more efficient way to get the news? Perhaps watch a very condensed news program or get your news via the internet?" While I have a large plasma TV at home, it is no longer connected to satellite, cable or any kind of antenna. I use my television exclusively for movies and I'm very selective about what I watch as I am starting to realize how precious time is when you start getting older. None of us are going to live forever. I choose to watch documentaries (where I can learn something), educational or biographical films (that inspire me), or shows that will simply make me laugh. All the other information I want to get updated on (news, weather, politics, etc.) I can quickly read or watch with a few clicks of my mouse and I don't have to sit through all the extra commercials! A quick story about also focusing too much on daily news via the traditional newspaper I'd like to share that is relevant. Eight years ago when I moved in to my apartment complex, almost half of the 40+ residents here got the newspaper delivered. Over time (with all the news now being available on-line), all of my neighbors stopped their newspaper delivery except for three ladies who get just the Sunday paper. One other lady in my apartment complex still gets two newspapers delivered every day: The Los Angeles Times and The Los Angeles Daily News. I know this because whenever I'm not traveling, I'll bring both of her papers from the front entrance and deliver them to her door. Just like the television news programs, shocking, horrific headlines help sell newspapers and just glancing at them for too long gets me depressed and upset. It seems like every other day there is a new embezzlement story from an L.A. city official or local politician. In some of these cases, corrupt individuals have embezzled or stolen millions of dollars! And we wonder why our taxes in California are so high? Perhaps all of my other neighbors decided to save time and money by stopping their home delivery, or perhaps they too were tired of being greeted in the morning with all the terrible headlines? My guess if they also choose to get their news on-line and selectively read the stories that interest them. At any rate, I find it interesting that the one lady who buries herself in both newspapers for several hours each day does not seem quite as chipper as the other neighbors when I run into her. Coincidence? Perhaps, but I'm not taking any chances, and as mentioned I cut off my 'boob tube' and selectively screen all the news I take in every day. There are many positive, inspiring stories in the world and so many exciting things to focus on, if you just look in the right places!

ACTION ITEM 34.0

Put a pen and paper by your television and log exactly how much time you spend watching TV. If you're averaging more than two hours per day, set a goal to cut out one show, or reduce your time in front of the 'boob tube' by at least 30 minutes per day. You'll be amazed what you will be able to do with all those extra hours each week! Perhaps read a book, exercise, cook a healthy meal, or spend more time with your family and loved ones.

Chapter 35.
'Program' Your Mind

Hopefully you now understand the importance of the 'Mind-Body' connection. To take advantage of this phenomenon, there are two important daily habits you can do to 'Program' your mind to help make you feel happier, healthier and more fulfilled: 1) Dedicate Time Each Day For Yourself. Most happy, successful people I know don't just *hope* each day is going to work out perfectly for them. This group of happy, successful people I studied spend 15 to 30 minutes each day for themselves. Uber successful, fulfilled people like Tony Robbins may even spend up to an hour preparing themselves for a successful day. Tony calls this time his 'Hour of Power' and includes a powerful technique he calls 'priming' which he does every single morning. The very successful and world-renowned Dr. Deepak Chopra wakes up at 4:00 am and mediates every day for almost two hours. This is not time for your spouse, your kids, or work related issues, but quiet time for *you* to meditate, reflect, and ask empowering questions. This focused time is spent reflecting on what you are grateful for in your life. If you're going through some current challenges (we all do from time to time), perhaps ask what you *could be* grateful for. Compared to so many people in other parts of the world, there is always something you can be thankful for if you ask the right questions. The best time to do this is first thing in the morning before you get distracted. My personal time starts at 4:30 am as soon as I wake up. At that time of the morning, I don't usually get any phone calls, IM's, text alerts, etc. and I do not turn on my computer. This is *my* time. I start this process by thinking of at least three things I'm grateful for in my life (one of which is being alive another day)! Don't be intimidated by needing to spend an hour on yourself every day, start off just spending just 15 or 30 minutes. Perhaps you spend five minutes thinking positive thoughts, praying or reminding yourself what you are grateful for. Then follow it up with a 15 to 20 minute walk or run around your neighborhood while you're focusing on your goals for the day. It doesn't matter whether you dedicate 15 minutes or an entire hour to focus on yourself each day, but you must spend a few minutes on *yourself* every day! For any parents reading this, don't see this as being selfish in any way. After you spend 30 minutes preparing yourself with positive thoughts and some exercise, you will have more energy and be in a better state to give more back to your children and spouse! 2) Pay Attention To and Transform Your Vocabulary. According to Robbins Research Institute, in 2001 there were approximately 750,000 words in the English language (today there are over 1 million words). Interestingly, there are only about 4,000 words that convey emotions. Approximately 3,600 of these words are used to describe *negative* feelings or emotions, while only about 400 are used to describe *positive* emotions. [35-1] Many of these emotional words whether written, read, spoken or simply heard can trigger feelings and emotions. Think for a moment about the people you encounter during the day and the simple response most people give when asked the most common greeting: "How are you doing today?". Most people answer: "Oh... I' m OK", "Can't complain", "I'm a little tired", "I'm surviving, but not enough coffee yet", "Getting by", or my favorite: "I'm hanging in there". Why not instill a simple new habit when a family member, roommate or co-worker asks how you're doing each morning, by cheerfully answering: "I'm doing great, thank you!", "Oh, fantastic", "Never been better!", or "Very well and you?". One of my favorite responses I learned from my brother Peter when someone asks how you're doing is to reply: "Second best day of my life!". That unique response changes people's state as they're so used to hearing negative or mundane responses to the common question. Often my response gets a follow up question: "Really... today is the second best day of your life? How is that?". My standard follow up response is: "Well, I'm expecting some really exciting news tomorrow, but I'm just an optimist!". This simple interaction usually puts a smile on the other person's face, puts a smile on my face, and often times both of us in this short exchange will get a chuckle. It's so simple (but vitally important) to think about the vocabulary you speak and the words you use including inside your head (your self-talk). If you make a conscious effort to transform your daily vocabulary, it will over time improve your health, happiness and outlook in life. This sounds very easy and overly simplistic, but trust me it works. If you start by removing just a few *negative* words from your daily vocabulary and replace them with *positive* emotional words, you <u>will</u> notice a difference in your energy and how you feel. This is one of the easiest habits you can implement today and quickly benefit from. Hopefully now you see and feel the mind-body connection and the importance of *programming* your mind so you can have more control of how your day is *going to go* rather than simply *going along with however your day goes*. It doesn't matter so much what happens to you during your day (we can't control everything that happens to us), but we *can* control how we handle and react to our day and the meaning of the moments in our day. Sometimes day-to-day life can be a little challenging. As Tony Robbins says: "See life as it is, but don't make it worse than it is." So how can you be one of those people who go through life with a smile on your face and seen to always be 'up' and enjoying life? I'm not talking about living in a fantasyland with a fake perma-grin on your face, but what daily habits can you instill to become someone who always seems positive? How can you become one of those people who seem to be productive and successful, yet make it look so easy?

Here are two examples of friends I asked to reveal their daily habits that help set their day up for success.

1) **Marla Grosslight** (an attractive, energetic lady who looks like she's in her late 40's, but admitted she is 61) is someone I run into from time to time around Hollywood. Every single time I see Marla - no exceptions, she has a huge smile on her face, is full of positive energy and always seems happy. Marla is one of those people you can't easily describe, but there's such an aura of positive, warm energy that you want to be around her. I interviewed Marla to find out exactly how she starts her day. Here's her secret routine every morning..."First of all, I want to ensure I get a good night's sleep, so I program my phone to 'do not disturb' mode (outside of my close family members), so I won't get any texts, tweets, calls, etc. during the night. When the alarm goes off, I gently roll out of bed and head to the kitchen where my coffee maker is set up. I grab a cup of coffee and curl back into bed for my 'quiet time' of 10 to 15 minutes". Marla explained to me her daily mantra where she says her grateful prayers. It's a very short (but important) list of people and things in her life she's thankful

for. This includes saying a blessing for the health and well being of her husband, her children and her grandson and anyone else who might need a prayer. Sometimes she'll say a short prayer for close friends who are sick, healing or going through some challenges. Marla then switches gears and thinks for a moment or two about what she is hoping for in the near future and thinking about what she wants to manifest in her life. After Marla gets out of bed (for good) to get ready for her day, she rarely turns on the daily news, which she explains, "has become so negative the way the media tends to dwell on and spin all the recent tragedies". If Marla needs to catch any important news, she'll have the TV on, but muted so she only catches the news that she needs (like a traffic update) before leaving her house. Her program of choice in the morning is watching the light, fun humor of Andy Cohen. When Marla finally leaves her house, she has another habit of always leaving plenty of time to get into L.A. (she lives about 15 miles north of Hollywood). If you're unfamiliar with the unpredictable traffic patters of the L.A. freeways, one morning it could be a 25-minute commute, the next morning it could be over an hour drive to work. Marla finds that allowing plenty of extra time minimizes any possible stress and with her favorite 'book on tape', she sets herself up for an enjoyable ride to whatever movie studio she's working at that day!

2) Monroe Mann is a truly unstoppable, energetic, 'Renaissance' gentleman in his 30's and a force to be reckoned with. Monroe is a proud army veteran who has lived in multiple countries around the world, speaks four different languages, and is a successful entrepreneur, a practicing attorney, and holds a doctorate in psychology. In addition to speaking and teaching, Monroe coaches and mentors successful people to achieve their wildest dreams. He has written almost a dozen books (some of which have become Amazon Best Sellers) and in his spare time he sings and produces music videos and movies! I know a little about Monroe's excellent habits from reading some of his books including one of my favorites: Time Zen. I was lucky enough to catch up with Monroe for a few minutes after his weekly Chinese class and before a business meeting in Manhattan (he telecommutes to Shanghai to improve his fluent Mandarin). Here's some insight into how Monroe (the uber-achiever) attacks each day..."The first thing I do every morning is glance at my phone. I don't necessarily respond to texts or return phone calls (unless they are urgent matters), but mainly to check on my clients, quickly scan the news events of the day on the Yahoo, Fox, and BBC new apps. I then jump right in to my 'To Do' list and that is where the daily magic happens." Backtracking a bit, understand that Monroe is so busy, he doesn't want to jump into just anything or get pulled in different directions like most people at the start of their day. Monroe programs his mind the night before. He types up a very specific To Do list for the following day, so he doesn't have to think about hitting each day running... he starts off in a full sprint. It's very important to note that this is *not* your normal To Do list. Monroe doesn't put items like laundry, dry cleaning, or paying bills on his daily list. He assumes those items will get done subconsciously, unless you're a strange person who wants to risk your power and phone getting cut off, or you don't mind wearing smelly, stained clothes. In all seriousness, the To Do list Monroe creates each night aligns with his goals and dreams. This process Monroe uses (as is the case with most successful, healthy, and happy people) takes no more than 5 to 10 minutes each night and keeps him on track to get what he really wants out of his life. This process also clears Monroe's mind, which helps him sleep better and allows his subconscious mind to drift towards his lofty dreams and ambitions. Monroe adds: "My mind is always working, and in the event I ever wake up in the middle of the night with a great idea or a solution for one of my many projects or clients (which does happen), I have a notepad and/or Siri on the nightstand near my bed to capture any ideas, which then allows me to quickly get back to sleep". Once again, Monroe's list is not a standard list of things he 'has' to do every day. Monroe's list is full of specific action items that he '*chooses*' to do each day that tie in to his goals, dreams and ambitions for the long road ahead. Some of these items might only take 5 to 10 minutes, but for every item on his list, he advances closer towards his long-term dreams while enjoying the process along the way. By 'chunking' his actions into smaller bits of time (like writing a rough draft of an introduction vs. trying to sit down and write an entire book), Monroe gets a lot more accomplished, feels constant momentum, and keeps his energy level up. This daily process that Monroe 'programs' the night before allows him to hit the ground running full speed in the morning and stay focused on what is important to *him*. Monroe's nightly process (which you can use also) really helps him avoid the many distractions we all face us in the modern world. For more free tips and great advice from Monroe, you can follow him on his YouTube channel www.YouTube.com/monroemann, join his network of winners at www.BreakDiving.com, or read more about Monroe and his many projects at www.MonroeMannLaw.com. Just like you feed your body with nutrients, it's vitally important to feed your minds like Marla and Monroe do. If you don't, our current society will program it for you through media and advertising.

Let me give you a specific example what happened over time to my mother several years ago with some bad habits she acquired over time. A few years ago I made my annual trip back to New Jersey to visit my mother and the rest of the family for Christmas. Although I communicate with my mother via the phone, email, etc. on a regular basis, this was the first time I'd seen her in person in a year. I noticed that she looked a little older (you often notice changes of people if there's been a time lapse), but what was most shocking to me was that while she still had faith in God, she had lost faith in almost everything and everybody else and was not as cheerful and upbeat as she used to be (part of this was related to health issues which can sap the energy out of anyone). The first day I got home, I noticed she was worried sick about the 'worst recession ever', the 'looming bank crisis', the 'horrific wars in the Middle East', the 'crumbling education system', etc. After visiting her for about a week and being immersed in her environment, I figured out the problem was all the bad 'programming' she was installing in her mind each day. This was her ritual most mornings:

1) Get out of bed early in the morning (often it would be dark) as my Mom is usually an early riser. Like most people, my mother has a standard clock radio with an alarm - not a pleasant sound to wake up to.

2) Turn on the television to watch and listen to all the news.

3) Go downstairs and get a cup of coffee.

4) Turn on one of the morning talk radio shows. Normally around the holidays, a large portion of these shows are ranting about politics with the recent elections and current events including the wars in Afghanistan and Iraq.

5) While making a sugary breakfast (juice drink, yogurt, toast & jelly, etc.), she would watch the morning news switching back and forth between different networks. Most of the news is extremely negative taking about the latest Wall Street scandal, the most recent U.S. corporation to file bankruptcy, the thousands of manufacturing jobs lost, the skyrocketing foreclosure rates, the local war hero who just committed suicide yesterday, the obesity epidemic, and the exponential growth of ADD and ADHD of our kids attending the growing number of failing schools. The most positive story might be a warning to make sure you don't eat any of the local vegetables, which could be tainted by Salmonella or a report to be careful about the rising toxicity in the local water supply!

6) As my mom would be getting ready for breakfast, she'd start reading the local newspaper, which had awful headlines covering the local politician who just got caught cheating on his wife with a prostitute while embezzling funds from a local charity.

Of course the back section of the paper has the obituaries, which was a must read section even if she didn't know any of the people who passed away that day. This all transpired in the first two hours of each day! What kind of state do you think all of this left my mother (or anyone else for that matter)? This quick story I share is in no way to pick on my mother, as I used to have similar habits many years ago and I was not a very optimistic or sunny person in the morning. In fact, I really didn't really get 'on a roll' until lunchtime when I used to go for a plate of barbeque chicken wings, curly French fries, and free refills of Coke with my good friend Bill Barnes. After some good old-fashioned barbeque and a few large Cokes, Bill and I would be ready to hit the phones for the rest of the day calling our customers when we both worked at Xerox. Bill was an awesome guy who I miss dearly, since a few years ago he also died from cancer. Being great friends with Bill and seeing the grief on his wife's face at his funeral and the sadness his young daughter went through was awful. This was one of the first wake up calls that I should start eating a healthier diet and also find a better way to start off my days. Anyway, getting back to the story of my mother, does this sound familiar? Like somebody *you* know very well? This 'programming' that too many of us allow as an everyday habit is not the best way to start your day! I firmly believe a big part of how people start their day is how they *program*, themselves and their minds. Do they watch and listen to all the negative news stories each morning? Or do they *program* themselves like Marla and Monroe do? What I love about getting news now from the internet is I can pick and choose what stories I want to read quickly without having to sit through all the other negative news stories. Being informed each day, doesn't have to mean losing your faith in humanity! My mother has since changed her daily morning rituals and is much happier and more optimistic.

A quick disclosure: my mother, Marla and Monroe admit they're not happy, full of boundless energy, or successful 100% of the time. Of course *nobody* is! In fact part of the juice in life are the occasional ups and downs, or the change of the 'four seasons'. Life would be boring is you were stuck on the beach with 365 days a year of sunlight and you never saw any clouds and never had any rain or thunderstorms. The variety in life is part of what makes it interesting and the reason we appreciate victories, celebrations, achievements and milestones. When you look at life from a different perspective (like being truly grateful), you can start appreciating and enjoying the little things in life, like how green the grass is, how a little flower just opened up on your walk to work, listening to a song bird signing his tunes, maybe noticing the beautiful and massive clouds rolling in for a rain or snow storm. We all know people who are millionaires (or at least well off) and seem to have all the material possessions they desire, a family who loves them, yet some of these people are *not* happy. We all know people who appear stressed or anxious, while others who seem to have very little stress are more relaxed and enjoy the moments in life. Why leave your emotional state (your happiness, health, personal fulfillment) to chance? The only way I know to be a better, healthier, happier, more successful person is to *program* your mind each and every day. I hope you do too!

ACTION ITEM 35.0

Think about one word you use on a regular basis that has a *negative* or *neutral* emotion to it, and replace that word with a *positive* or *empowering* one. For example: if every day when people ask how you're doing and your response is: "Oh... I'm OK", replace that with: "I'm doing great, thank you." By simply replacing one negative word or phrase for

an entire week with a positive one, you'll quickly see and feel the impact that your vocabulary can have!

Chapter 36.
Conclusion: The 'Three Secrets' to Great Health

As mentioned, over ten years ago I became intrigued with the 3 to 5% of the people who approached the Medco (later the Express Scripts) table after my presentations who were taking _no_ prescriptions. This very small group (the "Super Healthy 4%") exuded excellent health... they stood tall, had great skin, usually had a big smile, and proudly proclaimed that they took _no_ medications at all. Some even bragged they'd never even taken an aspirin. These incredibly healthy individuals were usually not in the free flu-shot line (at the table next to me), yet they claimed to never get the flu or sick like many of their co-workers. I consider myself very healthy, but I really wanted to know their secrets, especially within the many retiree groups I've worked where I often see people in their 70's, 80's who look amazing. It's almost expected (and certainly common) today when people reach 65 or retire in this country, they need to take prescription drugs on a daily basis. Inside the pharmaceutical industry, we call these 'maintenance' drugs and doctors often prescribe them for blood pressure, cholesterol, diabetes, thyroid, allergies, etc. The number of people on prescription drugs has skyrocketed the past five years almost as fast as the retail price hikes (and co-pays) for the many unfortunate folks who need to take pills every day.

Over the past 10 years since I started tracking numbers, I normally come up with a 3 to 5% figure for the people who take no prescriptions and stand out as being exceptionally healthy. However, that percentage of healthy people the past two years has been shrinking. While these are imperfect surveys I'm doing, I've worked a few fairs recently where 99% of a specific retiree population at that fair is taking some kind of prescriptions! Once again, these statistics I'm sharing are NOT perfect, but I'm sharing them to simply show a possible trend (that I'm seeing first hand) where more people are taking prescriptions and less people seem to be in perfect health. On October 30th, 2014 I flew to a San Francisco health benefits fair hosted by a large corporation that was having an open enrollment meeting for their employees and their recent retirees. Out of 603 people who came to my table that day, only 4 were *not* taking any prescriptions! To me this is tragic, but without further delay, let me get to the good news and share the 'Three Big Secrets' these select healthy people all had in common:

SECRET # 1) They Moved Their Body every single day. A few people went to the gym on a regular basis, but most did not 'work out', and very few in this group were exercise fanatics. Many did not even call it 'exercise'. But they all moved their body on a daily basis. Some pet owners took their dogs on long walks twice a day, others walked 3 to 5 miles around their neighborhood every day, rain or shine. Other folks worked in their garden or yard for at least an hour each day, 5 to 6 times each week. A few seniors enjoyed yoga or Tai Chi several times each week. It didn't matter how these healthy, drug free people moved their bodies, what was important was that they all shared this simple daily habit of moving their bodies or walking every single day (no exceptions). Some walked to the farmer's market, others down the street to their neighbors, to the post office, etc. They all understood that a daily walk, bike ride, playing outdoors with their grandchildren, working in the yard, etc. was critically important and also made them feel better.

SECRET # 2) They had a Healthy Diet. I will clarify as *fairly* healthy, as many were not vegans, vegetarians, or fanatics on counting calories, or pushing away a slice of pumpkin pie on Thanksgiving, or even adverse to celebrating with a cocktail now and then. Several of these people indulged in sweets, meats, or fast food, BUT did so in moderation. The longest living people (and all the individuals from the small % of super healthy folks) I interviewed for this book including several in their 80's and 90's had a diet of mostly vegetables and fruits, and a small amount of meats, processed or fast foods (if at all). As mentioned, these healthy folks indulged in desserts from time to time, enjoyed wine or cocktails on occasion, even lit up cigars when a new great grandchild arrived. I believe that not being too vigilant about rare indulgences kept these people from not stressing out - which leads to the final secret all of these super healthy people had in common.

SECRET # 3) A Positive Attitude. Every one of these people who visited my table were optimists who saw the glass as 'full' or at least 'half-full'. To quote several of them with their own words: "I don't worry about things I can't control." "It doesn't do me any good to sweat the small stuff" or my favorite: "If you're still living, why not simply enjoy life and have some fun every day?". This positive attitude has really rubbed off on me over the years and thanks to these super healthy, positive people, I always felt better after our conversations about health and vitality. After a typical health fair where on average 96 out of 100 people ask me questions about their prescription drug lists or ailments, it always makes my day to engage with the 4 or 5 healthy, positive, prescription free role models I normally saw each day! These three secrets might seem overly simplistic, and might even be a let-down if you were expecting some more profound, technical secrets, but if you take a little time to really apply these secrets every day (and make them daily Habits), I promise that over time you will see improved health, have more energy and feel better than you ever have before!

A final note to make the changes you want in your health. I've worked with over 500 people who've made dramatic improvements in their health, most starting off with the 7-Day "Alkalize & Energize" cleanse. It is critically important that you need to want to change and own the responsibility YOURSELF. Coaches are great, but in the end YOU have to make some of the small lifestyle changes in your diet, daily exercise and attitude yourself. Nobody else can make the changes for you. Ironically not even all of the people at the Health Benefit Fairs you may attend. I can't tell you how many 'professionals' and 'experts' I've seen at health fairs who are who are not fit and healthy themselves! I've seen gym membership directors who set up their table and talk to people about getting fit and signing them up for gym memberships, when they themselves are not in shape! This past year I was at a health fair for large client in California and the Registered Nurse and the Physician Assistant at the table next to me were obese and one of them was actually sick. These ladies took blood pressure, measured pulses and gave other tests and then giving 'one on one' health advice. These two 'wellness consultants' then gave out Cheetos and candy bars to everyone who came by their table as seen in the photo below! Just as there are some major flaws in our current health care system - of which I've outlined solutions to YOU in this book, the health benefits fair model is not perfect and I have a lot of great ideas and solutions on how to fix that as well. But that will be saved for a different book I'm writing specifically for the human resource managers and health benefits coordinators. But that's another story!

ACTION ITEM 36.0

Take the step today to start implementing one of these 3 'Secrets' and make it a daily habit. Make today the day you decide to go for a 30-minute walk during your lunch hour. (By the way, you can still return phone calls while you're walking). Or perhaps on your way home, you pick up extra vegetables, sprouts, nuts, or fruits and make tonight's meal a healthier one? Perhaps you spend 30 minutes today reading and savoring some inspiring quotes. Over time, you'll appreciate these 'Secrets' and become addicted to them as your daily habits!

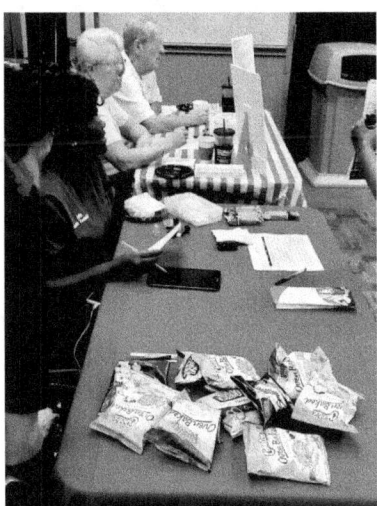

Ideas to improve Health Benefit
fairs coming in my next book!

<u>BONUS SECTION: Three Additional Health Tips</u>

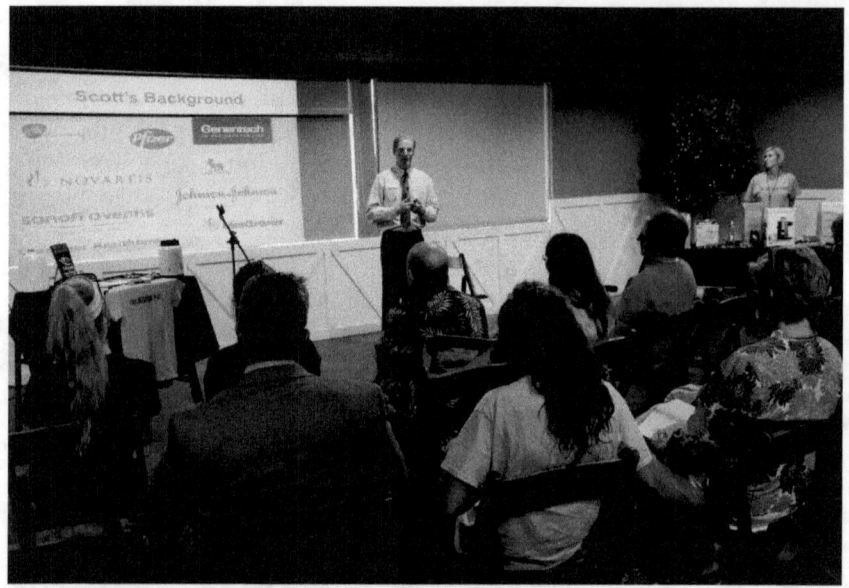

The author speaking on "The HEALTH Pill" national tour
giving additional Health Tips!
(photo by Tom Zapcic photography)

BONUS Chapter 1.
25 Tips for a Great Night's Sleep!

If you study the most productive, successful, and happy people, they usually don't sleep 8 or 9 hours every night. Most successful people I know sleep 5 to 7 hours each night (certainly not more than 8), but their *real secret* is they get a quality, restful sleep. I have a lot going in my life right now including writing several books, three different films in production and/or development, along with my day job(s) of coaching, speaking, training and acting not to mention quite a bit of travel. For me I like to get at least six hours of sleep a night (6 to 7 hours is ideal for me), but everyone is different. The most important thing about sleep is not only how many hours you sleep, but *how well* you sleep! I'll take six hours of restful, non-stop sleep over eight hours of intermittent or poor quality sleep every night. Here are a few habits I've developed over the last two decades that allow me to sleep like a baby almost every night. I'm confident many of these tips will help you get a better night's sleep as well:

1) Start With a Good Bed. Some people prefer a very stiff bed, while other people prefer a softer mattress. Just make sure that whatever you're sleeping on offers good support. You don't have to spend a fortune on your bed, but if you still have that second hand $50 mattress from college, it's time to upgrade!

2) Use a Small Pillow. This should be common sense, but I talk to people with neck or back pain and one of the first questions I ask is: "How many pillows do you have?" If you look at the slight curvature of the human spine, that should demonstrate that you shouldn't have two or three huge pillows jacked up underneath your head! This actually puts a kink in your neck and can partially close the airflow through your trachea (windpipe). I sleep either flat on my back with no pillow (with my back and neck totally straight) or on my side with one very small, soft pillow. You do not want to jack your neck up too high as it will be uncomfortable. When I sleep on my side I'll use one small pillow, which aligns my head and neck perfectly with my spine. In addition to washing your sheets on a regular basis, make sure you wash your pillowcase each week also and replace your pillow(s) every 2 to 3 years as dust mites and other allergens can accumulate inside older pillows. For people with severe dust allergies, you may consider getting special dust covers to put around your pillow and inside of your regular pillowcase. These help make a difference.

3) Be Careful When You Nap. If you ever take short naps, make sure to nap early in the day. You certainly don't want to a nap in the late afternoon or early evening. Napping too late in the day will have an adverse effect later on at night when you're trying to get a restful sleep.

4) Avoid Large, Late Dinners. As a general rule you don't want to eat a late dinner and you certainly don't want to eat any large meal 2 to 3 hours before you go to sleep. While breakfast should be the largest meal, your dinner should be the smallest meal of the day so that you're not taxing your stomach and digestive system all night long.

5) No Late-night Snacks. Healthy snacks like fruit, veggies are best, but ideally you don't want to eat anything within 1 to 2 hours of your bedtime.

6) Avoid Liquids (including water) at Least One Hour Before Bedtime. Remember the human bladder is only so big. People wonder why they wake up and have to pee several times during the night. One additional note: if you do wake up, one of your first instincts is to drink a few sips of water, as you may be very thirsty. Resist the urge and that will help you get back to sleep more quickly.

7) Limit Alcohol as it Can be a Double-edged Sword. Some people claim that one glass of wine at (or after) dinner will make them sleep better, but any more than one drink can make you restless during the night, due to your body trying to rid itself of toxins.

8) No Caffeine or Stimulants Past Mid-afternoon. You don't want to drink any coffee, tea or anything else with caffeine or stimulants more than 4 to 5 hours before you go to bed. No need to explain further; this should be common sense.

9) No Evening Exercise! While a yoga class in the late afternoon or a walk after dinner is fine, you don't want to do any major exercise (like a two hour gym workout or aerobics class) a few hours before retiring for bed. Any serious exercise like running or working out with weights should ideally be done first thing in the morning or by mid-afternoon. You don't want to stimulate your metabolism and energize your body close to your bedtime. Do you ever wonder why young kids who are playing and running around for hours right before bed, can't immediately get to sleep? Once again, it's best to exercise in the morning.

10) Wind Down. Everyone's habits for winding down are different, but I enjoy a movie after dinner or sometimes a good book. Perhaps some nice classical or jazz music and certainly not music with a fast EDM beat. I save that for the mornings. Cap the evening off with anything that helps you relax, wind down and get ready for bed.

11) Reading Rules. After you brush and floss your teeth, etc. and you've done everything else to get ready for bed, reading is a great ritual. However, you don't want to read any material that's too heavy, disturbing, or scary right before your head hits the pillow. Also you don't want to be reading from a brightly lit screen from your computer, iPad, smartphone, or any other back-lit device which will not allow your body to stimulate melatonin (your natural sleep aid). It's better to read a traditional paper book with the light shining away from your eyes, or use a Kindle or Nook, which don't have the 'back-lit' effect shining at your eyeballs right before bedtime.

12) Nightly Rituals. Did you have rituals when you were a kid, or if you have children now do you have certain rituals you practice with them? Like reading a bedtime story, getting on your knees and saying a prayer, or simply making a wish for a happy tomorrow? If you don't have nightly rituals, it's time to get back in this habit. Whether it's reading a book, saying a prayer, or simply recalling three things during the day that you're grateful for (something I do every night). You can also visualize or forecast three great things you want to happen tomorrow.

13) Unplug and Disconnect! Unless you need to check an urgent, time sensitive e-mail for work, you're better off not being on your computer, tablet or smartphone for at least 30 minutes before going to bed. This should be your time to 'wind down'. Even social media sites like Facebook or Twitter can keep your mind engaged long after you log off, so it's best to just say no.

14) Don't Let Your Pet(s) Push You Around! If you have pets, you might allow them to sleep in your bed and I wouldn't dare try and talk you out of that if that's your ritual. However I draw the line with this next rule. If your dog, cat, guinea pig, or any other animal in the middle of the night steals the covers, or drapes over your arm or leg (to the point where it's uncomfortable for you to sleep or get back to sleep), push your pet off the bed or pull back the covers. As much as you love your animals, it's more important for you to get a good night's sleep than your pet. This might seem cruel at 3:00 am to elbow your furry friend off the bed, but you'll be a much better pet owner if you get a good night's sleep. And remember, while you're working all the next day, your dog or cat can catch up on their sleeping all day long!

15) Keep a Consistent Sleep Schedule. Many of us have different work commitments or events. You may have a late dinner, an office party, a family activity, etc. but other than those special occasions, do your best to maintain a consistent and regular sleep schedule. I usually retire fairly early (before 10:00 pm), because I wake up every morning at 4:30 am. Being consistent also means waking up the same time on the weekends. I've found it better to catch up with a catnap if needed, rather than changing my sleep pattern back-and-forth like a yo-yo. Consistency is the key for a good night sleep.

16) Take a Warm Bath or Shower. Of course if you're dirty or hot and sweaty, you should take a bath or a shower before you go to sleep anyway, but make sure it's warm enough, so that it's comfortable and relaxing. Taking a cold bath or shower is better in the morning if you really want to wake up and jump start your metabolism.

17) Clean the Air. I have an air ionizer and purifier as well as flowers and plants in my bedroom, which clean the air and provide fresh oxygen. These small machines are totally silent, but work wonders! You can also try essential oils like lavender, which may help you sleep better.

18) Make Your Room Dark and Quiet. Before retiring to bed, I close my door and pull my shades tight. If you live in a noisy house or an apartment, I recommend placing a towel underneath your door jam as another preventative measure from possibly waking up from a family member or roommate in your house coming home late, getting up in the middle the night, or waking up before you do. The quieter it is inside your bedroom, the less likely you'll be disturbed.

19) Cool Your Bedroom. It helps you sleep when you have your bedroom at room temperature or slightly below room temperature. If you live in a very hot climate (I used to live in Florida where it was expensive to turn down the thermostat too low), I recommend getting a fan as a gentle breeze will not only be pleasant, but will also cool your body and allow you to sleep better without breaking your bank account.

20) Set Three Alarms. People think I'm crazy when I explain this, but this is important for me being in the entertainment business, as I often have to be on set by 6:00 or 7:00 am. Just like any job, there's no excuse for being late. I have one alarm clock plugged into the wall, a battery powered alarm clock (in case the power goes out), and an alarm on my cell phone. With these three alarms (I always double check that they're all set), I've never had anxiety or concerns about waking up in time for over 15 years. I have total peace of mind that at least one of my three alarm clocks will wake me up.

21) Take Notes. Keep a Pen and Note Pad by Your Bedside. Being in a creative Industry, I never want to miss a great idea that might pop into my head after I lie down to sleep. For you, it might be a work related issue or something you have to do the next day that you don't want to forget. If you have a small notepad and a pen handy, you can jot down your thoughts and completely clear your mind, so that you can go back to sleep quickly. Another option is to have a small voice recorder on your nightstand close to your bed, or simply ask for Siri to take a note.

22) Turn Your Text and Twitter Alerts Off or to Silent. You don't need your cell phone beeping or flashing during the night for the hours you're sleeping. This is common sense. Unless it's an emergency, you don't need possible distractions to wake you up during the night. If there's a real emergency, people will normally ring your telephone 2 to 3 times or until you pick up.

23) Stretch Out the Tension. When I lie down at night I take a few deep breaths, stretch my back and torso and my arms and legs. Sometimes if I've had a really stressful day, I'll gently crack my neck and back joints. Whatever I can do to stretch and release tension along with taking a few deep breaths is a good thing, which helps me relax and get to sleep easier.

24) Avoid Prescription or Over the Counter Sleeping Pills. After you embrace some of the habits I've outlined above, most people should be getting a more restful sleep without the need for sleeping pills. If you ever feel the need to take a pill, try all-natural Melatonin.

25) Breathe Freely. For anybody who snores and has trouble sleeping, look into a CPAP (Continuous Positive Airway Pressure) machine. This is a treatment that uses mild air pressure to keep your airways open and delivers amazing results with several friends I've spoken with who now use one to get a restful sleep. Another great tool is the 'Breathe Right' nasal strips if you need help keeping your nasal passages clear all night. These strips are sold at pharmacies and most super markets. A final thought - if you've ever had a night when you're tossing and turning and just can't get to sleep. Get out of bed and read for a while. That will often do the trick and then get back into bed when your body eventually feels tired.

ACTION ITEM B.1
Implement at least 2 or 3 of these Tips above <u>tonight</u> to get on the path to a more restful sleep!

BONUS Chapter 2.
**5 Travel Tips to Stay Healthy
and Energetic on the Road**

When I used to travel for Medco and now for Express Scripts, I can literally be on the road for two months of the year every fall when companies, schools and organizations hold their open enrollment Health Benefit Fairs. I used to come up with all kinds of excuses why I couldn't exercise enough or eat healthy. I'd come up with excuses like: "It's 11:00 pm and the only airport restaurant open is serving fast food" or "I can only find soft drinks and sugary snacks at the convenience store since it's midnight" or "Everything in the hotel is closed, except for the vending machines" and my favorite excuse I used to use: "I've been traveling since 5:00 am and it's now after midnight, so I just don't have time to work out". I used to believe all of those excuses, but I figured several years ago after I wrote my first health book that I should get creative and find ways to be healthy and stay energetic even when traveling. So here are a few tips I've used over the years that have made a huge difference in my health, my energy levels, and my ability to get a great night's sleep even in an unfamiliar hotel room bed:

1) Book an Upstairs Hotel Room Instead of One on the Ground Floor. Always choose a top floor when available. Do you remember the 'NET' chapter about creating an easy opportunity to walk up and down stairs? By booking yourself on the second or third floor (or better yet a higher floor), you give yourself the opportunity to walk up and down stairs when you check in, go down to the lobby, have a meal, any time you leave the hotel, and finally when you check out. Of course almost every hotel has a fitness center these days, but I always ask for a higher floor when booking my reservations.

2) Pack Using a Check List. I created a checklist on my computer and also a hard copy sheet I printed out called my 'Travel List'. I make sure to double check this list before every trip to ensure I pack my running shoes, athletic shorts, T-shirts, a few extra pairs of athletic socks, a jump rope and/or an athletic exercise band. None of this gear takes up much room in my suitcase, but it ensures that I always have gear to run, walk, work out, etc. Anywhere I travel, my athletic exercise band is one of my favorites. It takes up almost no room in my suitcase, yet I can exercise my ankles, calves, knees, etc. when I'm sitting on an airplane for many hours, or if I'm stuck working on my computer for a long time in my hotel room.

3) Utlilize Layovers and Rest Stops. If I have a layover in an airport for even 20 minutes, I'll take that time to speed walk all around the airport terminal between the different gates. If I have an important phone call to return, I can still make that call while I'm walking around. The last thing my body needs after sitting on a plane for three hours is to sit down at my next gate for another hour! If I'm driving long distances between clients and I take a rest room break, I don't just sit down and have a meal, I will make sure to make a phone call or have a light snack while also walking around for at least 5 or 10 minutes and get some fresh air. A brisk walk also helps keep me awake and alert if I'm doing a longer road trip over five hours. Another trick I do when doing long distance driving trips (more than 3 hours behind the wheel) is I always pack a small back massager in my travel bag. I got a small plastic one at the dollar store and when I'm in the driver's seat, I simply place the back massaging tool between my back and the car seat. By moving positions in the car seat or adjusting my back, I get an excellent massage for almost every single part of my back and shoulders the same time I'm driving. I did this last week on a road trip up to the Oroville, CA Hospital (a 7 hour drive from LA) and not only did it make my trip more enjoyable, but by massaging all the different pressure points of my back, neck, and shoulders, it stimulated more blood and oxygen flow so that I never got tired the whole trip!

4) Plan Healthy Drinks and Meals. The most important thing I pack is my refillable water bottle. When I fly, I'm not a big fan of paying $5.00 for a bottle of water in the airport gift shop, so I always look for a water fountain or a water filling station right after I go through TSA security. Hydrating is very important especially when you're flying at high altitudes or traveling to a dry destination like Las

Vegas. I also pack my own homemade trail mix, which includes almonds, cashews, peanuts, raisins, and cranberries. This is a perfect, nutritious and portable snack. I admit that finding a healthy meal at airports or highway road stops is a little challenging. However, you can usually find a salad if you look around, which is a safe and healthy bet. If I'm limited to fast food chains, I'll usually choose a Subway Veggie sandwich on wheat bread or have the Subway artist make a special salad. My safety net (and this has saved me countless times) is Amazing Greens Superfood in travel sleeves. I can tear open a single sleeve and dump ½ the sleeve's green powder into my large water bottle and shake. Voilà... I have instant nutrition and energy anytime! By the way, I'm not a coffee drinker, but I have to share a healthier alternative to regular coffee, which also comes in travel sleeves for any road warrior coffee drinkers out there. Valentus SlimROAST coffee is an all-natural, non-GMO, dark Italian roast with no chemicals, ginseng and only 4g of sugar. I asked several family members and friends to try out a few of the Valentus coffee travel sleeves while on the road and they all loved the taste and the convenience. If you'd like try some go to: www.YouSeeResults.com.

5) Tips for a Better Sleep While Traveling. Many people get anxious when traveling that they may not wake up for their morning meeting, catch their early flight, etc. so here are a few suggestions. Make sure you schedule three different wake up calls: the old fashioned front desk 'wake-up' call, the hotel room alarm clock, and the alarm on your cell phone. Also keep in mind the different time zones... if you fly west and go out to dinner at 8:00 pm, remember that it's really 11:00 pm for your east coast time clock! Don't stay out too late your first night and give your body's internal time clock a break! Another travel tip is to minimize strange noises in your hotel room that might interrupt your sleep. Since most hotels now have refrigerators in the room, you don't want to risk that loud clunking noise of the compressor kicking on and off multiple times during the night. Unless you sleep in the kitchen at your own home, this is NOT a natural noise that anybody is used to. Since I don't use the refrigerator in my hotel rooms, I open up the refrigerator door and turn the thermostat all the way off. On other units that don't have a thermostat, I simply unplug the refrigerator. If you decide to use the refrigerator, I'd suggest stuffing a few towels around the unit, so that you at least muffle the noisy compressor when it kicks on. A few final tips, when I arrive at my hotel I park far away from the entrance, so I can get in a brief walk. Then, the first thing I do after I check in, is ask where the fitness center is. First of all, I want to know where the fitness center is located, but I also want to refill my water bottle from the water cooler or water fountain that most fitness rooms provide. I may only work out once a day, but I go in and out of the fitness room 6 or 7 times each day refilling my water bottle. I could always go to the front desk and purchase a bottled water for $3 or $4, but even when I'm on an expense report, I still feel funny spending that much money to buy water, when I can drink free water right down the hallway. I hope you try out and enjoy a few of these travel tips.

Happy travels!

ACTION ITEM B2.0

The next time you travel, bring a refillable water bottle. Not only is it good to super hydrate with water, but if you drink enough you'll be less tempted to order a sugary, unhealthy beverage often found in airports and rest stops!

BONUS Chapter 3.
13 Tips to Boost Your Energy!

Most people have ambitions and dreams to grow, contribute, spend time with their family, significant others, etc. or at least they used to. The truth is every successful, happy person I know doesn't come home from their eight-hour work day and plop on the couch to watch TV for 2 to 3 hours. They usually work longer hours, wake up super early and often set aside extra time in the evenings or their weekends to focus what they want or what they feel is important in life. All of this takes time, but most importantly it takes extra ENERGY! A few of these tips may have been covered already in the book, but below are twelve extra tips I've discovered over the years to boost your own energy:

1) Move Your Body for at Least 20 Minutes Every Morning. I don't always have time super early in the morning to go to the gym as I have to handle important e-mails, return phone calls to the east coast, do some writing, and still get out the door by 6:00 or 7:00 am most mornings to work on set, wherever that may be. Even when I have a very early call time, I make it a <u>priority</u> to spend at least 20 minutes doing some form of quick exercise to jump-start my metabolism. This morning at 4:30 am I cranked out some push ups, planks, leg lifts, sit-ups and jumping jacks. There are dozens of quick, easy exercises you can do in just 20 minutes, unless you would prefer to take a brief walk around the neighborhood, but exercise is the most important thing you can do to quickly boost your energy. I admit, I wasn't thrilled when I first instilled this habit over 10 years ago, but I kept this quote on my bedside table which motivated me (as I shared earlier in the book):

> "Sometimes I wake up in the morning and go Ahh...
> I don't want to work out! But I do anyway,
> because I'll always feel better afterwards.
> I have never once worked out and felt worse."
> - Alexandra Paul

You might know my good friend Alexandra Paul from the famous 'Baywatch' TV series that ran for over a decade. She still looks incredible many years later and her quote still inspires me to continue this daily habit first thing every morning. The other important reason to exercise first thing in the morning, is if you have a long day at work and you get home late and are dead tired, the last thing most people want to do is to work out. And if you don't work out, then you either have a guilt trip or justify your procrastination by telling yourself "I'll work out tomorrow". We all know that doesn't always happen. I promise that if you instill this habit of exercising in the morning for at least 1 to 2 weeks, you'll feel so much better during the day and have extra energy that you'll be addicted to this daily habit! By the way, if you're one of those people who work an unusual job working 3 to 4 days with longer hours (perhaps 10 to 12 hours each day), you can also quickly energize your body on your afternoon break. Walk up and down the stairs for 15 minutes, do 100 jumping jacks, or take a power walk outside instead of sitting down in the break room. As Tony Robbins always reminds me: "Motion creates emotion." If you want to instantly feel better and boost your energy, *move your body*!

2) Fill Your Tank With 'High Octane' Fuel. Most people wouldn't dream of putting regular gas in their car when the higher octane is recommended, yet for some reason we don't always think about what kind of fuel (healthy, natural energetic food) we put in our own bodies. First thing in the morning after your exercise, you want to put all-natural, healthy fuel in your body and avoid any sugary, processed or toxic foods. I mix up my breakfast every day to make it interesting, but I usually start my day with a healthy veggie-fruit smoothie I blend up in a few minutes and if need be, I can take my drink on the road during my daily commute. In this morning's smoothie I started with organic almond milk, ½ a cucumber, cilantro, ½ an avocado, two carrots, a banana, organic hemp protein powder and a little raw agave for sweetener. It was absolutely delicious and I now have this fuel that will give me several hours of energy to get through my busy morning. You've probably heard the old adage "Breakfast is the most important meal of the day" and it's true. The general rule of thumb that all doctors and nutritionists agree on is you want to eat more calories earlier in the day with breakfast being your largest, most important meal. A study at Boston University School of Medicine showed that French men and women who consume 57% of their daily calories before 2:00 pm are very active in the evening. Americans take in only 38% of their daily calories before 2:00 pm and have far less energy typically stumbling over to the couch to watch television until bedtime. [B3-1] A few other tips during the day (either at your office or home) include replacing your candy bowl with a fruit bowl, and instead of reaching for a sugary donut or a preservative laden, artificial muffin for a mid-morning or afternoon snack, try some home made trail mix. If you're a coffee drinker, try a green tea or a 'green' drink instead. Start thinking of the food you're putting in your body as fuel (or energy) and you will start to notice an increased, consistent energy level!

3) Hydrate. Re-read the water (hydration) chapter if you need a reminder on why having enough water is so critical to your overall energy as well as the proper functioning of your brain. Drinking just two large glasses of lemon water can have an immediate effect on your energy level! Another factoid from Dr. Darden (director of research for Nautilus Sports) you'll find helpful if you are ever hot and tired: "A gallon of ice-cold water requires more than 200 calories of heat energy to warm it to the core body temperature providing you with more energy for your life." [B3-2]

4) Create _'Your'_ _Time_ First! Living in today's high technology era puts more demands on us than ever before. It's not just people talking to you or calling you on the phone. It's the barrage of e-mails, texts, PM's, IM's, blogs, multiple social media outlets on multiple smart computer devices. It can get overwhelming at times which can deplete your own energy! People look at me strange when I turn my cell phone off sometimes, or if I refuse to go on my computer for several hours at a time, but I've learned that I need to recharge _me_ first. If I'm at a business meeting or connecting with a good friend, I focus all of my attention on the meeting or that person. If I miss a call, that's what voice-mail is for. If someone sends me a text message, I'll read that text and reply on _my_ time. As mentioned in a previous chapter, my golden rule in the morning is I don't check my e-mails, text messages, or voice-mails for at least two hours after I wake up. I've created *my* time. From 4:30 am until 5:00 am (when my schedule allows), I get into a state of gratitude just for being alive and healthy as so many friends and family members are not living, but I still am! From 5:00 am to 7:00 am, I then focus on my goals and dreams for the current year. Most often I'll write, edit, brainstorm new ideas and plans, etc. A few years ago, I used to wake up and look at my phone, check my e-mails, open up my LinkedIn or FaceBook accounts, etc. and I'd often get overwhelmed with other people demanding responses from me even though 99% of those were not urgent or even time sensitive. I used to feel overwhelmed, distracted and often tired before 9:00 am! Please understand, if I have a 5:00 am conference call with one of my producing partners on the east coast, or if I'm expecting an urgent e-mail, text or call, of course I'll look out for those, but otherwise I refuse to let my focus and plans for the day get distracted or altered. If you follow this rule of not letting *other* people's demands encroach on *your* day's plans for the first few hours of your day, you'll find more quality time for *you* and you'll also feel a bit more at ease and have more energy to handle *your* agenda!

5) Turn Up the Lights! I've read several books on sleep over the years and all the doctors and psychiatrists who studied sleep patterns agreed that darkness tends to diminish energy (it's better to sleep in a dark room), while bright light (like the sun) tends to stimulate more energy inside of you. People living close to the north or south poles (during their respective winters) where there is very little light during their extremely short days often purchase UV lights to create their own natural light source. In my office and in my bedroom I have a large China Ball light (you can purchase one on Amazon for about $10) that hangs from the ceiling. The bright light gets softly diffused everywhere in the room without any harsh shadows. It is a very pleasing light. In the summer time, I install a 75W LED bulb and in the winter time, I have a 300W bulb that throws off an incredible amount of light along with a bit of heat. This very bright light during the darker, winter months really helps me balance and maintain my energy.

6) Crank up the Music! It's amazing how hearing your favorite song can instantly change your state. Different music with different beats and tempos can stimulate and trigger your energy, or relax and minimize your energy those times when you want to relax or get ready for sleep. Whether you want to help boost your energy for a five-mile run or simply get your creative juices flowing in the morning, turn the music up! I listen to all kinds of music depending on my mood, but if you enter my office before 6:00 am, you'll probably hear some EDM tunes flowing out of my headphones while I'm jamming away on my computer keyboard.

7) Do What You Enjoy to Do. You often hear about extremely passionate musicians who work all night recording sessions to finish an album, or artists who hole up for several days working on their latest masterpiece. That passion, drive or energy comes from within, as these people enjoy what they do enough to sometimes work 12, 14 or 16 hours a day. If you're not lucky enough to be a rock star, at least try to get into a field or line of work that you would find enjoyable most of the time. It's never too late to transition to a different career or do something you would find a deeper meaning than just punching a time card for a few dollars. Life is short, so you might as well spend most of your waking hours doing something you at least enjoy. Or perhaps over time you can shift into a career where you are making a difference in the world. A side benefit of doing something you enjoy (or that has significant meaning) is that during your non-working hours, you won't be completely burned out from a job that you dislike.

8) Take a Break. The reason employers allow and encourage breaks is that taking breaks actually increases productivity. Whether you go to the water cooler, chat with a co-worker for five minutes, take a rest room break, or walk outside for a few minutes for some fresh air, taking a short break will give you more energy. The key to taking a break is to do something different than what you've been doing the last few hours. If you're standing on your feet all day at a busy convention or on a noisy assembly line, sit down for five minutes and embrace some silence. If you're sitting at a desk all day long, take a five-minute power walk down the hallway. The most important thing is to remind yourself to take a break. It might seem counterproductive and appear to waste valuable time during the day for breaks, but in reality by taking a few well-deserved breaks, you'll boost your energy and be *more* productive.

9) Cut the Caffeine and Sugar Addictions. There's no dispute that stimulants like caffeine and sugar can perk up your brain and your body which make you feel good for a certain amount of time. The problem is when the caffeine wears off and after the sugar is burned up, you can 'crash and burn' hard. By incorporating some of these other 'TIPS' and minimizing your caffeine and sugar intake, you will have longer lasting, more sustainable energy in the long run.

10) Program Your Supercomputer. The human brain is like a supercomputer and the thoughts inside your brain can take your energy levels as high as a kite or drop down to basement levels in an instant. Have you ever seen a video of a depressed person who finds out they just won the lottery? Or a completely happy person who gets the news that their closest loved one just died in a car accident? These are extreme examples, but I think you get the idea that there is a direct mind-body connection. So why not program your brain all day with positive, inspiring, energetic thoughts? You can read positive or interesting books, watch inspiring moves, repeat affirmations to yourself, speak incantations out loud, post enlightening messages or quotes around your office or house, or manage the vocabulary you speak every day. What ever you need to do to program your mind in a positive manner will directly effect your emotions and your energy levels.

11) Smile and Laugh! Take a look at this quote below:

"The average adult laughs 15 times a day;
the average child, more than 400 times."
- Martha Beck

Perhaps this is one of the reasons why kids often have more energy? I know for a fact if I go to a party where people are laughing it up, smiling and having a great time, not only do I want to stay at that party longer, but I can feel the positive energy. If I go to a party where everyone is complaining about something or gossiping about other people and the conversation is totally negative, I feel down. Don't be afraid to bring back some of the 'childish' behavior that many of us lost after entering adulthood. If you really want to get serious about this laughing matter try attending a Laughter Therapy seminar or sit in on a Laughter Yoga group in your city. I kid you not, they really exist and can be a lot of fun!

12) Don't Sweat the Small Stuff. Life is full of challenges, obstacles, and sometimes bad news. Take the news in, but don't dwell on it. Ask yourself: "Is there a message from what happened?" "Is there something I can learn from the challenge thrown at me?" There's usually a positive side to challenges and/or setbacks, even if you don't see it right way. One of my favorite questions I ask myself when I face a huge setback or get some disturbing news is: "What will this really mean in my life 10 years from now?" The reality is probably nothing! Once again, acknowledge and learn from your bad experiences, but don't sweat the small stuff that gets thrown your way. It's all part of life.

13) Straighten Up! I have a post-it note right next to my computer that reads: 'CHECK POSTURE!'. When you spend a few hours in front of your computer, it's an easy habit to fall into a downward gaze or develop poor posture. The combination of looking down and having slouched shoulders can drain your personal energy. In fact, poor posture can reduce the amount of oxygen you take into your lungs by more than 30% which is another reason why poor posture can reduce your energy! [B3-3] If that ever happens to me, I quickly see my post-it note which reminds me to straighten up, take a deep breath and get back to my goals for the day!

ACTION ITEM B3.0
Write down 3 things you can do to boost your energy now! Put on some music, do some jumping jacks, fix a 'green' drink, etc. If you can't think of anything, do yourself a favor and read the book Energy Addict. You'll find unlimited ways to live a more energetic life!

APPENDIX

7- Day "Alkalize & Energize!"
Cleanse notes:

Day 1 - 7: (Most people do 7 days, you can extend to 10 days if you wish.)

Day 2 - 3 (12 – 16 oz.) large glasses of alkaline, filtered water with lemon slices 1st thing in the am

1 (16 oz.) large glass of fresh cucumber, spinach, carrot, broccoli, juice for breakfast*

6 - 8 large glasses (or bottles) of alkaline, filtered water with lemon during the day

1 (16 oz.) large glass of fresh cucumber, spinach, kale, broccoli, juice for lunch if hungry

2 - 3 "Green" powder drinks* during the day for energy & nutrition.

1 small cup of raw, unsalted, all natural almonds (chewed completely before swallowing. This is a good snack w-protein & very alkaline).

1 - 2 Cups of "Green" Tea (with lemon for flavor – NO sugar, honey, Agave, or sweeteners of any kind)

1 (16 oz.) glass of celery, green squash, carrot, green pepper juice for dinner.

ADDITIONAL NOTES:
Do NOT eat any fruits or drink any fruit juice for 7 days as fruit has sugar (& any trace amount of sugar is acidic!)

You can mix different vegetables each day if you want. Try squash, zucchini, green beans, kale, asparagus, sprouts, spinach, etc.

Stay away from frozen, cooked, canned, or processed vegetables as they have less nutritional value & can be acidic.

Make sure you DON'T drink any store bought canned vegetable juice. V-8 and other brands are loaded with potassium chloride, sugar, magnesium, ascorbic acid, citric acid, added salt & lots of preservatives.

On **Day 5**, start drinking 2 - 3 glasses of Metamucil (with Psyllium husks) each day.

Your system should be completely cleaned out & detoxified by day 7.

*Fruit exception: you may use a ½ apple slice if needed in your vegetable juice for the first 2 – 3 days if the taste is too bitter.

*Fruit juice exception: you may add 1 – 2 oz. of apple juice into "Green" powdered drink along with your water if the first 2 – 3 days, if the taste is too bitter for you.

Quotes from Medical Experts:

"Up to 90% of diseases are due to improper functioning of the colon.... Of the 22,000 operations that I have performed, I have never found a single normal colon."

- Dr. John Harvey Kellogg

"Every physician should realize that the intestinal toxemia (poisons) are the most important primary and contributing causes of many disorders and diseases of the human body."

- Gastroenterologist, Dr. Anthony Bassler

"More than 65 different health challenges are caused by a toxic colon."

- The Royal Society of Medicine of Great Britain

7-Day "Alkalize & Energize!"

Common Mistakes:

Common Mistake:	Typical Example(s):	Explanation:
1a. "Cheating"	Eating a banana or having 1 glass of wine (these are usually influenced by friends or family who are unhealthy themselves).	Even a small amount of sugar (in fruit or alcohol) will not allow your body to fully alkalize.
1b. Lying to Yourself	Telling yourself that 1 piece of candy won't matter and you can make it up in the morning.	NA
2. Starvation Mode	Juicing only once a day.	If you don't get enough calories, your body will NOT drop weight, but instead retain that fat as a defense mechanism called "starvation mode".
3. Allowing an old habit to interfere	Smoking	Any smoke you put into your mouth or lungs is acidic.
4. Not "alkalizing" enough.	In addition to juicing, you should be drinking at least 2 – 3 "Green" Drinks each day (either powdered "Green" drink, or wheat grass).	It takes 4 parts alkalinity to counter 1 part acidity. During the 7-day cleanse, you need to super-alkalize your system to allow your body to start losing weight.
5. Too much extreme physical exercise!	Sneaking into the gym one day to lift weights, doing wind sprints, or a long endurance run.	Almost nobody believes or understands this, but this is TRUE. Any extreme exercise will create **lactic acid** in your system and then you are back to square one.
6a. Not getting enough	Besides walking up the stairs in their	The key to start removing acids and

exercise.	house or walking down the hallway at work, most people do NOT get real daily exercise anymore.	toxins from your body is muscle movement and aerobic exercise. Walking several miles, doing a gentle 30 – 45 minute hike, going on a long bicycle ride, doing a yoga class, etc. will.
6b. Taking in more calories than you are burning.	Taking in 2,000 calories each day and only burning 1,900.	Common sense – if you are not exercising enough to burn off the calories you are intaking each day, these excess calories will be stored as fat. This is normally how people gain weight in the first place!
7. Juicing late at night or right before you go to bed.	NA	Common sense would dictate NOT to give your body lots of alkaline nutrition when you are trying to wind down & go to sleep.
8. Irregular sleep pattern	Waking up & going to bed at different times every day.	A regular sleep pattern will allow your body cells to rest & recover each day. Not getting enough sleep can make your body acidic.
9. Negative thoughts or stress.	This could even be ANY negative "vocabulary" that you use when speaking such as: "I am so stupid".	Just because you did 1 stupid thing, does not mean you are stupid!
10. Continuing to take vitamins, supplements, etc.	Do not take any supplements of vitamins unless your doctor says you must.	Vitamins and other supplements often have sugar, and other chemicals added to them. These 7 days you want to clean all of that out of your system!

Frequently Asked Questions (FAQ):

Q: What is the 7-Day "Alkalize & Energize!" Cleanse Program?
A: This is a 7-Day Liquid Cleanse that will "Alkalize & Energize" your body. We do not want to underestimate how much better you feel in just 7 days, but for any skeptics, we will provide 'before' & 'after' photos of both authors who have done this many times before. The 500+ other people who have also done this cleanse as well ALL had dramatic results & took photos they kept for themselves. The U.S. leads all developed countries with over 66% of the population overweight & 30% of the population morbidly obese! If you are part of these statistics, this program will help.

Q: What's the Best Time to Get Started?
A: Right Now! Most people in the U.S. have built up toxins & poisons in their body through added chemicals, 3rd generation pesticides, antibiotics, steroids, super growth hormones, excess sugars, additives & preservatives that were not in our foods just 25 years ago. The only time we do NOT recommend to start this would be over the Holidays being surrounded by all the sweets, sugar treats, excessive food, coffee & alcohol.

Q: What do I Need to Get Started?
A:
1. A Vegetable Juicer – you can borrow one, or else you can find one for $40 - $75 at Wal-Mart or about $25 on Craig's List or e-Bay will get you a nice used one. A juicer (which separates the juice from all the pulp) is not to be confused with a blender!
2. "Green" Powdered Drink – you can buy from a health food store, Vitamin Shoppe, etc. A medium size container will last you a few months & should cost between $15 - $25. It is important to make sure this powder is only "Greens" with NO added sugar, corn syrup, fructose, or any additives. Also, it's best not to buy any Green drink that has any berries or fruit added – if it does, make sure it does not have more than 1g of sugar.
3. Alkaline Water – if you're not purchasing alkaline water or have a Kangen™ type of water system, we recommend

you use a filtration system that mounts on your kitchen faucet, or an inexpensive Britta™ type of water pitcher-filter. You should add lemon slices to your glass or pitcher, which will alkalize the water. Also add 1 ice cube to each glass of alkaline water when you drink. The ice cube will slowly change from a solid state to a liquid state, giving you a slight bit of energy.

4. Fresh Vegetables you can find in your local farmer's market or grocery store. Buy organic when possible. If you cannot afford organic, make sure you carefully wash all vegetables before juicing.

5. Fresh Lemons to add to your water. Do NOT add store bought lemon juice!

6. Green Tea - especially if you are a coffee drinker & feel you need a little caffeine. You may substitute "green" tea for coffee this week. Make sure the tea you get is all natural with has no added sugars or flavorings.

7. Psyllium Husk (most common brand is Metamucil). A small container of powdered Psyllium Husk is more than enough as you are only taking this the last 2 days of your cleanse.

8. Raw Almonds – a great alkaline protein snack for this week. Get a small bag or can of almonds & make sure there are raw & NOT roasted or salted & there is no sugar or added flavors.

Q: Will I Get Hungry at all or Have Food Cravings?

A: You might have some minor cravings the 1st or 2nd day if you have Yeast & Candida in your system. The candida feed on sugars, processed foods and acids, which you will be eliminating. If you do the program exactly as we recommend & drink LOTS of alkaline water and powdered "Green" drink in between your meals, you should not feel any hunger after the 2nd day. Part of the hunger is "psychological" with not eating solid foods and missing the act of eating. If you should feel a little hungry, drink a tall glass or bottle of water, or another bottle of Green drink. It is critical to have a water and/or "Green" drink in front of you at ALL times. This week you will be super-hydrating your system.

Q: How I Can Get Enough Nutrition From one 16 - 20 oz. Glass of Juice compared to the Large Portions of Food I'm used to Eating?
A: Since the vegetable juice you drink is all-natural and loaded with natural nutrition, vitamins, proteins, & minerals your body can easily digest & quickly assimilate, this will provide as much (if not more energy) than a huge meal that your body can not fully utilize. This is common sense.

Q: What if I Have a Business Lunch or a Planned Outing with Food?
A: There is nothing wrong with ordering a glass of lemon water or an Green tea with lemon and explaining you are not hungry. If it's too awkward at a big business meeting to not eat anything, you may have a bowl of split pea soup or a green salad with NO dressing. For dressing you can add some lemon juice and a dash of ground black pepper. Make sure the salad has no fruits in it (no raisins, cranberries, apples, etc. as these fruits contain lots of sugar). If you feel compelled to eat a salad one day for a business lunch, etc. you do NOT need to "fall off the wagon" and stop your cleanse! Just make sure you chew the lettuce, cucumbers, brochili, etc. very slowly & completely before you swallow. As you continue chewing, the more pepsin & renin (digestive enzymes) will be released to help break the salad down closer towards a liquid state.

Q: What Are the Main Rules (and any Foods to Avoid) for these 7 Days?
A: You're going to eat (actually drink) all ALKALINE foods. Mostly green vegetables, sprouts, etc. and powdered Green drink that you mix with water. You must avoid all acidic foods (processed refined foods, meats, dairy, fruits, bread, pasta, sugars, etc.) to cleanse & detox your system.

Q: Why Can't I Eat Fruit... I Heard Fruit was a Healthy Food?
A: Fruits are healthy foods, but most fruits are loaded with sugar. To properly "alkalize" you do not want to consume any fruits or fruit juices (and all these sugars) for the 1st 7 days while you're on this cleanse. You may be tempted to eat one banana, an apple, or an avocado, but you must NOT eat any fruit for these 7 days.

Q: Will I Really Feel That Much Better?

A: Yes! We've asked all the other people who have done this program to describe in a journal how they feel after the 5th or 6th day. Here is how some of our friends & family have described their health and energy after just a few days: "energized, alive, super-charged, new vitality, vigor, stamina, bouncing off the walls, excited, happy, renewed, rejuvenated, happy, healthy, like the fountain of youth!"

Q: I'm on Prescription Drugs & Take Several "Over the Counter" Medications. Should I Stop Taking Them?

A: You are not alone. 48% of all Americans now take prescription drugs on a regular basis and almost 90% of people over the age of age of 70 take some kind of prescription drugs! Most of this is due to an acidic diet & lack of exercise. You should NOT change your regiment of prescriptions unless you talk to your doctor. Many people who have done this program have gotten off most of their prescriptions & medications. Some over time have completely stopped taking all their medications! Remember that it may take several weeks or months to get off your medications, & you should always consult with your doctor, as your body gets more alkaline & back towards a state of perfect health.

Q: Can I Stop Taking Vitamins and Store Bought Supplements?

A: Unless your doctor has specifically told you to take certain vitamins or supplements, you should not take these during the 7-Day cleanse. The natural vitamins, minerals, and overall nutrition you'll get from the vegetable juice & green drink will be more than what your body needs. The reality in many cases the store bought vitamins contain sorbitol & sucralose (added sugars) & the supplements often just give you expensive urine.

Q: Why Should I Have a Journal or Make Notes?

A: In addition to taking a photo & weighing yourself before you start & after Day 7 (these "before" & "after" photos will be show some of your physical results), you'll want to write down a few notes each day on how you feel & what signals your body is telling you. We had one gentleman who had a large cut that scabbed up & while on the cleanse and it completely healed in just 3 days. This was a person who was so acidic before it would take him 2 to 3 weeks for a cut to completely heal!

Q: What I Do After the 1st 7 Days?

A: Please call us & we can discuss which route you want to go. We've had some friends continue juicing for many months who have lost 60, even 100lbs!, but most importantly they feel better & healthier every single day. Other people prefer getting back to a solid-food diet & we can walk you through a plan where you can go back to a regular, healthy food diet. This a healthy "lifestyle" assuming that 80% of your food & drinks all natural & alkaline which will help you maintain the great health you should be feeling after just 7 days. The choice is yours.

Q: Why Do I Lose So Much Weight so Quickly?

A: Most people with a "western" diet (especially in the U.S.) eating lots of processed & refined foods loaded with sugars & meats, which are very acidic. To check your acidity before your cleanse, you can either have a blood test done, or get a simple pH strip test (sold at your local pharmacy) to test your ph level before you start. The main reason people in this country are obese (and there are millions of morbidly obese people in the U.S. today) is that their body's natural defense to extra acid is to store lots of fat. This extra fat protects your body including all the vital organs. In just a few days, when your body starts becoming more & more alkaline, you will start shedding pounds even without a lot of exercise. Every single person who has done this program has lost 1 – 4 lbs. each day!

Q: Why Can't I Do a Lot of Physical Exercise?

A: We recommend NOT lifting heavy weights, doing wind sprints, or super long runs as these activities will produce lactic acid in your system. Daily exercise such as walking, biking, hiking, or even moderate jogging are fine & recommended. Any kind of yoga, stretching or exercise where you doing deep diaphragmatic breathing is excellent as these breathing exercises will activate your lymphatic system to help clean out the toxins in your body. Sitting in a steam room or a sauna for a limited time is also fine as this will help toxins escape your body.

**Q: At Certain Times During the Day I Feel Tired...
Is this Normal?**
A: Most likely you're not drinking enough Green Drink (which is pure alkaline energy). We've also noticed (with time capture cameras) people sitting motionless at their computers for 3 - 4 hours at a time. If your only body part moving is your mouse finger, it's no surprise you will feel tired! Make a point of standing up every 30 minutes & taking a quick break every hour or two. This is common sense! A great tip to make sure you do this is to set the timer on your cell phone for 90 minutes or write your break time on a post-it note. To keep your energy level up, you NEED to get up at least every 90 minutes to get more water, take a bathroom break, etc. On Day or 6 or 7 (when the Metamucil is working through your colon), you may feel a little tired until you discharge. Some people in our studies on Day 7 have lost 5 – 10lbs! This is painless, and you should feel amazing after that bulk of toxins & fecal matter has completely passed.

Q: Are You Sponsored by Any Company(s) Products?
A: No. The author of this book lost many close relatives & friends the past few years to cancer & disease. This information is being shared to help others reclaim the excellent health everyone deserves. Although heart disease, arthritis, high cholesterol, obesity, acid reflux, muscle & joint pains are "common" for people in the U.S., this was not "normal" 50 years ago. The author has worked for Medco and Express Scripts for many years & will tell you from personal experience the amount of prescription drugs that even young people are now taking (people in their 20s in 30s) has increasing dramatically the last 3 years. The U.S. Government & private companies burdened with these expensive health care costs are finally realizing that a better solution to start getting their employees healthier is though better diet & exercise.

Q: I've Been Doing the Cleanse for 3 Days and Haven't Lost Any Weight?
A: See the attached table, but there are four (4) main reasons:
        1) You are cheating with a piece of fruit or a glass of fruit juice. Even a few raisins or cranberries have extra

sugar in them. You can NOT have any sugar for these 7 days, as excess sugar will convert to acid.

2) You are not having 3 meals (or drinks) per day. If you try and "cheat" and don't take nutritional calories in every 5 – 6 hours, your body will go into "starvation" mode and will not release any of it's extra fat. This is why most low calorie or depriving diets don't work.

3) You are drinking too much vegetable juice. If you are drinking very large amounts of juice at one time (20 – 25 ounces is too much), not only will you have expensive urine, but your body may store some of this excess nutrition in the form of fat.

4) You worked out too hard! Both authors made this mistake by lifting heavy weights during a cleanse. Neither lost any weight those days, and in fact Scott gained 1.4 lbs. in one day due to the fact that an intense workout like sprinting or lifting weights creates lots of "lactic acid" in your. That lactic acid in turn signals your body to keep storing fat to protect your vital organs from this new acid in your system.

Q: Any last Minute Tips?
A: Yes. Do not put your water pitcher in the refrigerator. You'll be drinking so much water each day (2 - 4 liters) & you don't want to chill your core body too much. It's better to drink room temperature water. However, we do recommend putting 1 small ice cube into each large glass of water you drink. This won't chill the water that much, but as the cube transforms from a "solid" state to a "liquid" state of energy, it will help energize you! Also, you should stop drinking water at least 1 hour before you go to bed. Drinking an extra 2 – 3 large glasses of water right before going to sleep may cause you to use the rest room during the night. Also if you notice the 3rd or 4th day your feet smell, or you have a little body odor, that is natural. That smell is the toxins (which have built up in your body over many years) finally escaping!

Q: How Do I Continue After the Cleanse?
A: If you stop the cleanse after 7 days, 10 days, or 30 days, you then want to transition to a healthy lifestyle diet which is sustainable LONG-TERM. Simply ensure that 80 – 90% of your diet (all foods, beverages, snacks, etc.) is alkaline. The easiest way is to make sure that most of your

diet is made up of vegetables and a limited amount of fruits. There are several charts including a great one by Dr. Theodore Baroody in his book Alkalize or Die, but here is a very comprehensive chart:

www.acidalkalinediet.com/Alkaline-Foods-Chart.htm.

As long as MOST (as mentioned in our books 80 to 90%) of your diet is alkaline and healthy, you should still be able to have that slice of birthday cake, pumpkin pie, or chocolate chip cookie now and then on special occasions.

Q: Can You Share Some Recipes or Examples of What You Eat?
A: I strongly suggest you invest in a healthy (alkaline) cookbook, or get one from your local library. Instead of turning this into a full-blown recipe book, we simply wanted to educate you and point you in the right direction. With that said, here is a sample of what Scott (the author) eats on a typical day:

Breakfast:
(an hour or so after several glasses of alkaline water):
Vegetable-Fruit Smoothie. In a blender add 1 cup of organic almond milk, 2 large leaf clusters of Kale, 1 carrot, ½ of an avocado, 1 banana, 1 tablespoon of Hemp protein powder, 1 teaspoon of organic Agave sweetener, a splash of pure vanilla extract and 2 ice cubes. Fill the top of the blender with filtered water depending on how many people the drink is serving.

Lunch:
Large salad with lots of greens and alkaline vegetables. You can sprinkle in a small handful of cranberries, raisins, and blueberries if desired. I like to spring ground walnuts, pecans, or almonds on top for extra protein. For dressing only use a tiny amount of extra virgin olive oil & balsamic vinegar and then add lots of fresh squeezed lemon juice on top as well for some zest.
A great soup combo to go with this salad is split-pea soup, with which you can add in minced celery, mushrooms, or spinach for extra protein.
For a drink, have a nice glass of **Green Tea** sweetened with lemon or a little Agave.

Dinner:
Black Bean Taco Soup. 1 can of natural black beans (no sugar or sodium added). Sliced red onions, mushrooms, roma tomatoes, diced scallions, 1 avocado and simmer. Add soup over organic, unsalted taco chips. Add a dash of black pepper if desired and sprinkle basil and parsley flakes on top and serve warm.

For a drink try a combination $1/3^{rd}$ apple juice and $1/3^{rd}$ cranberry-pomegranate juice with the top $1/3^{rd}$ of the glass topped off with water. The water will slightly dilute the high sugar content found in the fruit juices.

Early evening snack:
1 glass of **red wine with some green snap-peas,** or you can try a small bowl piece of **fresh, ripe fruit**.

Reference Notes

1-1 www.sustainabletable.org, "Corn and Soy" May 12, 2015

1-2 TIME Magazine, "Microbiologist on a Mission" - Louise Slaughter March 27, 2015

1-3 USA Today, "Health", March 14, 2015

1-4 www.diabetes.org, "The Cost of Diabetes" May 12, 2015

3-1 www.MedicalDaily.com, "Microwaves Are Bad For You: 5 Reasons Why Microwave Oven Cooking Is Harming Your Health" - Lizette Borreli, August 10, 2013

5-1 www.YahooNews.com, "Food". March 30, 2015

5-2 Nemours Marketing, Inc., "Informal Study on Meats served on Los Angeles area Film & Television production sets" (2009 - 2014)

5-3 www.FactoryFarming.com, "Overview of the Animal Factory"

5-4 www.cdc.gov, (Centers for Disease Control and Prevention) "Heart Disease Fact Sheet / Data & Statistics November 30, 2015

5-5 www.cancercouncil.com, - "The Cancer Council Report"

6-1 www.MotherJones.com, "USDA Ruffles Feathers With New Poultry Inspection Policy".- Philpott, T. April 24, 2013.

6-2 The Guardian, "If Consumers Knew How Farmed Chickens Were Raised". April 24, 2016

7-1 www.MicrobeWiki.com, "Antibiotic Use for Farm Animals"

7-2 TIME Magazine, "Microbiologist on a Mission" - Louise Slaughter, April 27, 2015

[7-3] www.Healthline.com

[7-4] Business Insider, "The Disgusting Truth About Fish And Shrimp From Asian Farms" - Jennifer Welsh, October 23, 2012

[8-1] www.nutritionstudies.org "Frightening Facts About Milk", - Thomas Campbell, MD, October 31, 2014

[8-2] "Forks Over Knives", Monica Beach Productions, 2011

[8-3] LBN-News, May 1, 2015

[8-4] The China Study, - Dr. T. Colin Campbell, BenBella Books, 2004

[8-5] The China Study, - Dr. T. Colin Campbell, BenBella Books, 2004

[9-1] TIME Magazine, "Weight Issues", page 11. July 9, 2012

[9-2] The pH Miracle: Balance Your Diet, Reclaim Your Health - Robert O. Young, PhD. and Shelley Redford Young, 2008

[10-1] www.Businessinsider.com, "American Per-Capita Sugar Consumption Hits 100 Pounds Per Year". - Henry Blodget, February 19, 2012.

[10-2] USA Today, "Youth Diabetes, Pre-diabetes Rates Soar". - Nanci Hellmich, May 20, 2012.

[12-1] www.GreenandJuicy.com, "Spotlight on Raw Foods: Living Energy for Living Bodies" November 28, 2010

[12-2] www.naturalnews.com, "Lavender and It's High Vibrational Frequency"

[14-1] The Daily Mail, "Only 1 in 100 Dieters Keeps the Weight Off." - Sean Poulter, May 14, 2016

[15-1] www.telegraph.co.uk, "Ancient Romans 'had Perfect Teeth' Thanks to Healthy Low-sugar Diet", October 4, 2015

16-1 p. 24 Living Skinny in Fat Genes, by Dr. Felicia Stoler, R.D. Pegasus Books, 2010

16-2 www.aarp.org/health "Fit and Fab at 50+: Tosca Reno" by Stacy Julien, December 29, 2014

18-1 www.GetHolisticHealth.com, "Woman Drinks Gallon of Water Every Day for Four Weeks and The Final Picture Results Are Shocking!" November 17, 2014

21-1 www.YahooNews.com, Health: "Obesity Trend in America" June 19, 2015

21-2 The Daily Mail, "Western Lifestyle to Blame for Soaring Breast Cancer Rates", August 9, 2010

21-3 The Journal of Nutrition, "Adolescent Obesity Increases Significantly in Second and Third Generation U.S. Immigrants", April 1998

21-4 US-China Today, "Obesity in China: Waistlines are Expanding Twice as Fast as GDP", April 8, 2011

22-1 Stanford News Report, July 21, 2004 "Obese Parents Increase Kids' Risk of Being Overweight."

23-1 "Get the Edge" audio program by Tony Robbins, Robbins Research International © 2000

24-1 www.FlowingData.com, "Who Spends the Most Years in Retirement?", Nathan Yau

24-2 The Independent, "A Daily Walk Can add Seven Years to Your Life" September 4, 2015

24-3 Bloomberg Business, "Kill Your Desk Chair and Start Standing" by Drake Bennett, June 28, 2012

25-1 CBS News, "OMG, You're Texting Your Way to Back Pain." - Jessica Firger, November 14, 2014

27-1 www.Merriam-Webster.com

29-1 www.Arthritis.org, "12 Benefits of Walking."

29-2 www.independent.co.uk, Health News: "A Daily Walk can add Seven Years to Your Life." August 30, 2015

31-1 Do These Things or You Will Die: 5 Secrets to a Long, Healthy, and Energetic Life! - Scott duPont, Nemours Publishing, 2013

31-2 Robbins Research, Institute. www.tonyrobbins.com

32-1 TIME Magazine, "Health" July 11, 2016 p.47

34-1 New York Daily News, "Average American Watches Five Hours of TV Per Day", David Hinckley March 5, 2014

34-2 "Lawyers and Settlements" January, 2007

34-3 Centers for Disease Control and Prevention, NCHS Data Brief Number 76, October, 2011

35-1 "The Power to Shape Your Destiny: Seven Strategies for Massive Results" by Tony Robbins. © 2001 Robbins Research International

B3.1 Energy Addict, Jon Gordon, Berkley Publishing, 2003 p. 23

B3.2 Energy Addict, Jon Gordon, Berkley Publishing, 2003 p. 37

B3.3 Energy Addict, Jon Gordon, Berkley Publishing, 2003 p. 58

Bibliography
(Recommended Reading):

The 30-Day Diabetes Miracle Cookbook, Bonnie House & Dianna Flemming, PhD, LDN, Perigee © 2008

Alkalize or Die, Dr. Theodore A. Baroody, Holographic Health Press ©1991

Alzheimers Disease: What if There Was a Cure?, Mary T. Neport, M.D. Basic Health Publications © 2011

A Smoothie a Day Keeps the Doctor Away, Chad Napier, CreateSpace © 2016

The Auschwitz Volunteer: Beyond Bravery, Captain Witold Pilecki, Aquila Polonica © 2012

Biomarkers – The 10 Keys to Prolonging Vitality, William Evans, M.D., Simon & Schuster © 1991

Breast Cancer – Beyond Convention, Mary Tagliferri, M.D. Atria Books © 2002

Cancer – Step Outside the Box Ty Bollinger © 2006

Childhood Cancer Survivors, Nancy Keene, O'Reilly © 2000

The Complete Encyclopedia of Natural Healing, Gary Null PhD. © 2005

Creating Health, Deepak Choprah, M.D., Houghton Mifflin © 1991

Curing Fatigue, David S. Bell, M.D. St. Martin's Press ©1993

Do These Things or You Will Die ...5 Secrets to a Long, Healthy, & Energetic Life, Scott duPont & Ronald Farnham, Nemours Publishing, Inc. © 2013

Energistics, Phyllis Paulette, Paperjacks © 1987
Fit for Life, Harvey and Marilyn Diamond, Warner Books ©1987

Food is Your Best Medicine, Henry G. Bieler, M.D., Random House, Inc. © 1966

The Food Revolution, by John Robbins, Conari Press © 2001

Forever Young, Dr. Nicholas Perricone, Atria Books © 2010

Fuel – The Energy You Need to Succeed, Wes Beavis, Powerborn © 2009.

The Gerson Therapy, Charlotte Gerson and Morton Walker, Kensington Publishing © 2001

Healing Foods, Patricia Hausman, Dell ©1989

Healing the Gerson Way, Charlotte Gerson and Beata Bishop, Totality Books © 2009.

It's My Life! I Can Change If I Want To, Richard D. Walker © 2011

Jamie's Food Revolution: Rediscover How to Cook Simple, Delicious, Affordable Meals, Jamie Oliver © 2011

Living Skinny in Fat Genes, Dr. Felicia Stoler, R.D.
Pegasus Books © 2010

May All Be Fed, John Robbins, Morrow © 1992

Natural Cures "They" Don't Want You To Know
About, Kevin Trudeau © 2006

The New Fit or Fat, Covert Bailey, Houghton Miiflin
Company © 1991

The Omnivore's Dilemma, Michael Pollan. © 2007

Our Toxic World, Doris J. Rapp, M.D., Environmental
Medical Research Foundation © 2004

The pH Miracle: Balance Your Diet, Reclaim Your
Health Robert O. Young, PhD. and Shelley Redford
Young. © 2008

Positive Energy, Judith Orloff, M.D., Harmony Books
© 2004

Real Age, Michael F. Roizen, M.D., Cliff Street Books
© 2000

The Relation of Alimentation and Disease, Dr. James
R. Salisbury © 1888

Reversing Fibromyalgia, Dr. Joe M. Elrod, Woodland
Publishing © 2002

Self Test Nutrition Guide, Dr. Cass Igram, Knowledge
House © 1994

Stand Tall: Every Woman's Guide to Preventing
Osteoporosis, Morris Notelovitz, Bantam Dell
Publishing Group © 1985

Surgery and Its Alternatives, Sandra McLanahan, M.D., Twin Stream Books © 2002

Tarascon Pocket Pharmacopedia, Jones & Bartlett © 2012

Think Better - Live Better, Joel Osteen, Faith Words © 2016

The Total Cancer Wellness Guide, Kim Thiboldeaux, BenBella Books © 2007

Toxemia Explained – The True Interpretation of the Cause of Disease J. H. Tilden, M. D., © 1935

The Ultimate Healing System: The Illustrated Guide to Muscle Testing & Nutrition, Gary Null PhD. © 1998
A Week in the Zone, Barry Sears, Ph.D. Harper Paperbacks © 2000

Walking with the Power, Dexter Clay, Black Eye World Publishing © 2004

Your Body's Many Cries for Water, F. Batmanghelidj, M.D., Global Health Solutions © 1997

Photo Credits

All photos are property of Nemours Marketing, Inc. or Scott duPont, Inc., unless listed otherwise underneath the photograph(s).

<u>100% TOTAL SATISFACTION GUARANTEE:</u>

If for ANY reason you are not 100% satisfied with the book, CD or DVD you purchased, just send the product back along with receipt (or proof of payment). We will gladly refund 100% of your money, no questions asked!

Nemours Marketing, Inc.
7531 Azurebrook Court
Winter Park, FL 32792
www.TheHealthPill.com
info@NemoursMarketing.com
Tel: (407) 738 - 1608